Pediatric Endocrinology for the House Officer

Dennis M. Styne, M.D.

Associate Professor of Pediatrics
Director, Pediatric Endocrinology Research Laboratory
University of California, Davis
Davis, California

With Contributions by
Matthew H. Connors M.D.

Associate Professor of Pediatrics
School of Medicine
University of California
Davis, CA
and
Russell W. Chesney, M.D.

Professor and Chairman
Department of Pediatrics
LeBonheur Children's Medical Center
Memphis, TN 38103

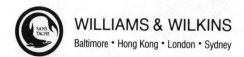

WILLIAMS & WILKINS

Baltimore • Hong Kong • London • Sydney

Editor: Nancy Collins
Associate Editor: Carol Eckhart
Copy Editor: Diane Castilaw
Design: JoAnne Janowiak
Illustration Planning: Wayne Hubbel
Production: Raymond E. Reter
Cover Design: Dan Pfisterer

Printed in the United States of America

Library of Congress Cataloging in Publication Data

Styne, Dennis M.
    Pediatric endocrinology for the house officer/Dennis M. Styne.
      p. cm.
    Includes bibliographies and index.
    ISBN 0-683-07937-9
    1. Pediatric endocrinology. I. Title.
    [DNLM: 1. Endocrine Diseases—in infancy & childhood. WS 330
S938p]
RJ418.S78 1988
618.92'4—dc19
DNLM/DLC
for Library of Congress

87-37125
CIP

88 89 90 91
2 3 4 5 6 7 8 9 10

This book is dedicated to my loving wife and children, Donna, Rachel, and Jonathan, who have supported me throughout this endeavour and so many others.

Preface

Since the informal birth of pediatric endocrinology in the late 1940's, with the clinical and biochemical observations of Dr. Lawson Wilkins at the Harriet Lane Home of Johns Hopkins University Medical School, a progression of over four academic generations of pediatric endocrinologists have advanced the field to its present importance in pediatrics. Progress in assay techniques, physiology, and molecular biology have brought the subspecialty to the point that the causes of most disorders are known and systematic approaches to their treatment are available. Pediatric endocrinology interfaces with all other aspects of pediatrics; any systemic disease can cause abnormalities of growth or pubertal development.

It is the intent of this book to provide a basic understanding of the disorders of the endocrine system that can occur in childhood and furnish a basic approach to the diagnosis and treatment of these disorders to students, house staff, and practicing physicians. The limitations of size preclude a complete discussion of the physiology upon which the approach to the patient is based, and we strongly encourage the reader to consult references supplied with the chapters to delve further into the pathophysiologic mechanisms of the diseases considered. Furthermore, although the strategies for evaluation of some of the conditions are straightforward, others will surely require consultation with a physician familiar with the field of pediatric endocrinology. For example, the diagnosis of a newborn with ambiguous genitalia and the approach to discussions with the parents are not to be undertaken by a novice. Further, variations in manifestations of some conditions and vagaries of laboratory results require individual attention when the patient does not present in a classic manner. The laboratory values furnished in this book are only to be used as a general guide; the standards of the laboratory being used should be considered. Drug dosages are also supplied as a guide; package inserts and pharmacists should be consulted for the latest recommendation in case of a change in suggested dosage.

The chapters are organized in a lecture format so that the book may be taken as a set of core presentations covering the basics of pediatric endocrinology. It is organized on the basis of endocrine systems with the closing chapters dealing with emergencies and laboratory tests in a multi-organ fashion. It is our hope that this volume proves a useful ready reference for the physician evaluating children with endocrine disorders.

Dennis Styne, M.D.

Acknowledgments

The facts in this book draw upon the teachings and writings of a legion of endocrinologists: the suggested readings credit a reasonable sample of these workers. Among them I must give particular credit to my mentors, Drs. Melvin M. Grumbach, Selna Kaplan and Felix Conte of the University of California, San Fransisco. At the University of California, Davis, Dr. Mark Wheeler was extremely helpful in proofreading and suggesting appropriate changes in the text while Sean Barry mastered the intricacies of word processing and laser printing. Thanks also go to the uncounted students and house-officers upon whom I sharpened my teaching techniques.

Contents

Chapter 1

Growth

Short stature is the most common complaint that brings a child to a pediatric endocrinologist. However, growth is a general indication of a child's health and growth abnormalities can herald the onset of non-endocrine systemic disease. The thrust of this chapter will be the evaluation of endocrine disorders, but all other chronic conditions should be ruled out before a sophisticated endocrine evaluation is started.

THE MEASUREMENT OF GROWTH

It cannot be overemphasized that *measurement of stature* is the cheapest procedure available in the pediatric office and the one most often incorrectly performed or not performed at all! Forgetting to measure a child is a serious mistake that limits the assessment of the health of the child. Further, if a growth deficiency is developing, the most important measure of the defect, the growth rate, cannot be assessed until an extra visit and measurement is obtained, at the cost of another three months or more. Also, because most systemic diseases can affect growth, the decrease in growth rate (an early indication of the onset of such a disease) would be missed. Incorrect measurements are responsible for numerous incorrect referrals for short stature and can obscure the effects of a medication meant to correct an abnormality of stature.

After the measurement is obtained, it must be displayed graphically on the *growth chart*. An abnormality of stature or growth is far more obvious on a graph than written as a number on the page. A decrease in growth rate in which the child "falls away from the curve" becomes obvious on the graph.

1

An accurate measurement of *infant length* is extremely difficult and always requires two adults. The child must be laid on a flat surface with a device that has one plate horizontal to the plane of the top of the child's head and another horizontal to the first in the plane of the child's feet. The two plates should be at a 90 degree angle to a ruler on which the child's height is read. No other method is usable; the worst method, unfortunately in common use, calls for an observer to make a mark on the paper covering the examining table at the foot of the child and another at the head so that the distance between the marks can be measured. It should be obvious that this technique will not eliminate parallax at the head and feet, that the paper is so flexible as to make the distance between the head and feet quite variable (if the paper crumples during the measuring procedure, the distance may vary even more), and that the movement of even a relatively quiet child will make such measurements useless.

The measurement of a patient more than two years old is done with the child standing. The switch from lying to *standing measurements* is responsible for a large number of inappropriate referrals due to the 1 to 2 cm decrease in height that occurs when switching from lying to standing; the type of measurement should be indicated on the chart next to the numerical measurement for children between two and four years old so that this mistake will not occur. Regrettably, it is necessary to caution the observer to measure the child with the child's shoes off; we have received numerous patient records with the child measured in shoes one time and without them another time, a condition which is guaranteed to cause 2 to 4 cm variation in height per visit. The device used to measure standing height must be a respectable variation of a *stadiometer*. Thus, the child must have the back to the wall or to a hard surface; the back is straight, and heels and back press posteriorly to the surface. The feet must be on a plane made of a hard surface, considered to be the bottom of the measurement; the top must be a hard plate completely horizontal to the plane of the feet, and the measurement must be read off a stationary ruler that is at right angles to the planes at the feet and head. A *Harpenden stadiometer* is the most accurate of such devices, but even a homemade device that follows the above guidelines should give accurate measurements. Unfortunately, the device attached to the common office scale is used in many pediatric offices. The plate at the top of the pole is rarely horizontal to the floor; without any way to straighten the patient's back, the child may slouch.

We strongly recommend making all measurements in the *metric system*. The tendency to round off numbers becomes problematic when an inch is the unit of measure; an inaccuracy of an inch or a half inch is a more serious error than a mistake of one or a half centimeter; remember that a half inch (1.25 cm) rounding error over a six month period can mean the difference between 4 cm/yr growth, which is abnormal, and 6.5 cm/yr, which is normal.

The *arm span* is measured from the outstretched middle fingertips while the patient is standing with the back to the wall and with the arms spread horizontally. The *upper to lower segment ratio* is measured from the top of the symphysis pubis to the floor as the lower segment. The upper segment is the height of the child minus the lower segment.

Skeletal development, or *bone age*, is more closely correlated with certain developmental landmarks than with chronological age in conditions of delayed or advanced development. The bone age is determined by an x-ray of the left hand and wrist as compared to the *Greulich and Pyle atlas*. The delay or advancement in bone age is expressed in standard deviations from the average reading for chronological age. Increased accuracy in the technique is accomplished by radiologists with the most practice; unfortunately, most general radiologists who are not associated with a pediatric center do not read many bone ages and their readings may not be quite correct. With a bone age over six years and an accurate determination of stature, final height can be predicted by the *Bailey-Pinneau table*s found at the end of the Greulich and Pyle atlas. The *RWT method* allows prediction in younger children of eventual adult height (see Appendix I).

ENDOCRINE FACTORS IN GROWTH

Growth hormone has a major effect on postnatal growth but probably has no role in prenatal growth. The release of growth hormone is stimulated by *growth hormone releasing factor* and inhibited by *somatostatin* or *growth hormone-release inhibitory factor*. Growth hormone has direct diabetogenic effects, but the growth promoting action of growth hormone is postulated to occur through *somatomedin* or *insulin-like growth factor (IGF)*. Growth hormone concentrations are low throughout most of the day in normal patients but rise at intervals, especially during the electroencephalogram stages 3 or 4 that occur soon after going to sleep. Thus, random growth hormone measurements rarely are revealing of abnormalities of secretion; only sequential measurements through a 12- or 24-hour period or measurements after the administration of a secretagogue are of interest. In growth hormone deficiency, the bone age development is delayed, whereas the upper to lower segment ratio is normal for bone age in contrast to hypothyroidism where bone age is severely delayed but the upper to lower segment ratio is quite increased due to lack of appropriate growth of the limbs in the absence of adequate thyroid hormone. Patients with untreated growth hormone deficiency have delay in the onset of puberty.

IGFs, or *somatomedins,* are produced in mesenchymal tissue throughout the body, but the major source of somatomedin is the liver. Somatomedins are thought to cause growth by attaching to receptors in the cartilage; somatomedins have mitogenic effects in most dividing cells in the body.

Insulin-like growth factor 1 (IGF-1) is the somatomedin most closely associated with growth. Plasma levels of IGF-1 fall in states of growth hormone deficiency and rise in growth hormone excess. IGF-1 is low in the neonate and rises slowly through childhood until a peak is reached during the pubertal period; values at this stage are in the acromegalic range. Except for this rise that occurs near the pubertal growth spurt, absolute plasma concentrations of IGF-1 are not closely related to growth rate. The major problems with the interpretation of IGF-1 concentrations are (a) the values in the first three years of postnatal life are close to or identical with those found in the hypopituitary state; (b) the values in constitutional delay in growth are appropriate for bone age rather than chronological age; and (c) in states of poor nutrition, a condition that by itself can cause poor growth, IGF-1 values are as low as those in a growth hormone deficient subject. Thus, the use of commercial IGF-1 tests must be tempered with caution in the diagnosis of growth deficiency.

Concentrations of *insulin-like growth factor 2 (IGF-2)* are decreased in growth hormone deficiency but not raised in growth hormone excess. Levels also may also be increased in patients with osteosarcoma.

While plasma IGF-1 concentrations may not be reliable in the diagnosis of growth hormone deficiency, the finding of low values of IGF-1 and IGF-2 has been stated to be quite reliable in pointing to the diagnosis.

Thyroid hormone is essential for postnatal growth but has little effect on fetal longitudinal growth. Thyroid hormone is also necessary for the secretion of growth hormone as hypothyroid patients may not respond to growth hormone stimulation tests. In the absence of adequate thyroid hormone, the patient has reduced limb growth, leading to a retarded or higher upper to lower segment ratio. Bone age development is also retarded in hypothyroidism. Usually puberty is delayed if thyroid hormone is decreased, but with profound hypothyroidism puberty may occur prematurely.

Sex steroids can advance growth, skeletal age, and pubertal development in the postnatal state. Gonadal steroids are essential for the pubertal growth spurt and are responsible for approximately one-half of the growth achieved during puberty. If excessive sex steroid concentrations are maintained for a long period, the epiphyses will fuse and the previously tall child will become a short adult.

Glucocorticoids are the most effective growth suppressors when encountered in excess; thus, Cushing syndrome due to endogenous or exogenous glucocorticoids can cause the cessation of growth and short stature. Decreased glucocorticoids will not affect growth.

Insulin in excess will increase growth rate in the fetus and after birth, for example in patients with insulinomas or islet cell hypertrophy. A deficiency of insulin will decrease growth because of the diabetic condition which will occur. Further, in the absence of insulin receptors, as in the leprechaun syndrome, fetal and postnatal growth will be poor.

Genetic factors are of obvious importance in growth. The correlation between midparental height and children's height can be used to adjust the position of a child on a growth chart. Therefore, a child at the fifth percentile of the growth chart who has short parents may in fact be closer to the tenth percentile when adjusted for midparental height. Standards for the adjustment of American children's heights are presented by Roche and standards for British children are presented by Tanner.

Nutrition is the most essential factor for growth and reproductive development. In the evaluation of children from developing countries it may be inappropriate to consider the parents' heights as they may have been subject to malnutrition during their growing years and may be inappropriately short while the child may benefit from better nutrition and have the opportunity to be taller than the parents. Voluntary decrease in nutrients or chronic disease can exert the same effect as economic malnutrition on decreasing growth. Thus, socioeconomic and psychosocial factors are important considerations in the interpretation of growth rate.

Chronic disease may decrease growth apart from its effects on decreasing nutritional intake. For example, the decrease in stature in children with juvenile rheumatoid arthritis is not necessarily nutritional.

Psychologic problems can affect growth either from a nutritional standpoint or through an endocrine effect. Psychosocial dwarfism is a temporary hypopituitary condition precipitated by abnormal

ABNORMALITIES OF GROWTH

Short Stature

Nonendocrine Causes

Constitutional delay in growth and adolescence (constitutional delay) is not a disease but a variation of normal development. After a normal birth length and weight, growth rate decreases during the first two years so that stature becomes shorter than average for age. In addition, bone age is delayed two standard deviations; the child is usually thin, and the growth rate is appropriate for the skeletal development. Thus the growth rate must be interpreted in terms of bone age rather than chronological age. If the patient has genetic short stature in addition to constitutional delay in growth, the degree of short stature may be so obvious that the patient will seek advice; if constitutional delay occurs in a child without genetic short stature, the degree of short stature may not stimulate a medical evaluation. There is often one parent or a sibling with a history of constitutional delay in the family history.

Patients with constitutional delay will enter puberty at a later age than their peers but appropriate for their bone age. The final height of such children may be normal or shorter than average according to conflicting studies. The predicted height of boys with significant delay in bone age may overestimate final adult height.

Genetic short stature refers to the child of shorter than average parents. These children are expected to reach a reduced final height.

Intrauterine growth-retarded (IUGR) infants are born with weights below the tenth percentile for their gestational age; for a full term baby this translates into a weight less than 2500 grams. These children remain small for their entire growing period and attain short adult heights. The patients are characteristically thin, have bone ages appropriate for chronological age, have a normal age of onset of puberty, and usually have a normal to low normal rate of growth.

Many syndromes have IUGR as a characteristic. Frequently encountered situations include *fetal alcohol syndrome* (also associated with microcephaly, short palpebral feature, epicanthal folds, small jaws and short philtrum of the lip, cardiac defects, and some delay in mental development), *maternal smoking, maternal drug abuse,* the dominantly inherited *Noonan syndrome* (with some characteristics reminiscent of Turner syndrome) and the sporadic *Russell Silver dwarfism* with clinodactyly (radial bending due to a triangular middle phalanx) of the fifth fingers, asymmetry of the extremities, and a triangular-shaped face.

Numerous syndromes including abnormal karyotypes will have short stature as one of their characteristics. *Turner syndrome* has absence or abnormalities of the X chromosome. There are many other karyotypic disorders with short stature as one component.

Other syndromes combine short stature and obesity, a combination that should awaken concern over an organic etiology for short stature as patients with exogenous obesity are usually tall for age. *Laurence-Moon-Biedel syndrome, Prader-Willi syndrome, pseudohypoparathyroidism* as well as *Cushing syndrome, hypothyroidism,* and *growth hormone deficiency* lead to short stature and obesity.

Chronic disease of any organ system can cause growth retardation, and any pediatrics textbook will have such cases on virtually every page. The onset of a chronic disease may even be dated by a decrease in the growth rate noted on a growth chart.

Malnutrition, a frequent cause of short stature, may be due to maternal neglect, poverty and lack of available food, neurologic impairment that decreases interest in food or causes inability to swallow it, malabsorption or even voluntary lack of food intake. Somatomedin may be decreased with any of these, and the unwary investigator may incorrectly consider that growth hormone deficiency is at fault.

"Failure to thrive" includes a wide variety of conditions in which an infant is not growing well. Usually, the weight is affected before and to a greater degree than the length or height; this is in contrast to the effects of hypothyroidism and growth hormone deficiency where weight is maintained but growth slows. These infants may have reflux, parents inexperienced in feeding infants, aberrant intrafamilial dynamics, and many other chronic conditions alluded to above.

Endocrine Causes of Short Stature

Growth Hormone Deficiency

Classic growth hormone deficiency has been found in approximately 1 in 4000 children in Scotland; the incidence in the United States may be lower, but even at one-half that estimate, growth hormone deficiency must be considered a common disease. When acquired growth hormone deficiency (such as that caused by head and neck irradiation used to treat children with cancer) is added in the equation, growth hormone deficiency must always be considered as a possible etiology in a patient with growth failure.

Idiopathic growth hormone deficiency is considered to be due to decreased hypothalamic GHRH in the majority of cases. Rarely patients are found without pituitary glands or somatotrophs. An increasing number of cases of short stature are attributed to partial lack of growth hormone. The dividing line between growth hormone deficiency and normal growth hormone secretion is becoming increasingly blurred.

Congenital growth hormone deficiency does not affect fetal growth, and the child has a normal birth length. Soon after birth, however, careful observation will indicate abnormally low growth rate. The patient will be obviously short for age by two to four years of age and the diagnosis often will be suggested at this point. Classic patients will have a cherubic appearance of chubbiness and a high-pitched voice due to a small larynx but adequate vocal ability to speak appropriately for chronological age. They appear precocious because their appearance suggests a younger age, but their speech and abilities suggest an older one. Males may have microphallus (stretched penis length less than 2.5 cm), especially if there is associated gonadotropin deficiency. Hypoglycemia may occur in the absence of the gluconeogenic growth hormone, which acts as an anti-insulin factor. If adrenocorticotropic hormone is also absent, more profound hypoglycemia is possible (cortisol also stimulates gluconeogenesis): in either situation there may be hypoglycemic seizures. The combination of *hypoglycemic seizures and normal birth length* should alert the observer of the possibility of neonatal hypopituitarism; if the patient is a male with microphallus or if there is optic hypoplasia, the diagnosis must be ruled out before any other condition is considered.

Midline defects ranging from cleft palate to encephalocele are associated with congenital hypopituitarism. Optic hypoplasia with any degree of visual impairment and usually with pendular nystagmus is a frequent indication of associated hypopituitarism. Absence of the septum pellucidum is found in 50% of patients with optic hypoplasia and pituitary impairment.

Breech delivery or indeed any type of neonatal head trauma are other associated historic findings in patients with congenital hypopituitarism.

Familial growth hormone deficiency may occur in autosomal recessive or dominant patterns or in an X-linked pattern. Kindreds are known that completely lack the gene for the production of growth hormone.

Laron dwarfism combines poor growth and high basal and stimulated growth hormone concentrations with low IGF concentrations and an absence of receptors for growth hormone; patients cannot respond to growth hormone administration with increased somatomedin concentrations.

Pygmies have normal growth hormone concentrations and normal IGF-1 but very low IGF-2 concentrations. They are of normal height until puberty but lack a pubertal growth spurt.

Biologically inactive growth hormone has been postulated as a cause of normal growth hormone concentrations measured by radioimmunoassay but the ability to respond to exogenous growth hormone administration: the true incidence of this disorder is unknown, and some patients identified as such may have "partial growth hormone deficiency."

Diagnosis of Growth Hormone Deficiency

The diagnosis of growth hormone deficiency has become more complex with increased knowledge of growth hormone physiology. Although there are certain times when growth hormone treatment may be beneficial without classic growth hormone deficiency, we will only deal with clear indications in this chapter.

Classic growth hormone deficiency is defined by the inability to raise growth hormone concentration above an accepted limit (generally 10 ng/ml in most laboratories) after two *stimulatory tests*. As mentioned above, the measurement of basal growth hormone concentrations is useless unless the timing is perfect and the sample is taken just as the patient is experiencing a spontaneous peak of growth hormone. Ten minutes after 10 minutes of vigorous *exercise* (almost to the point of exhaustion) normal children will raise their growth hormone in 80% of trials. Sequential samples at night may be taken in the hope that the peak that customarily occurs 90 minutes after the onset of sleep, but this method is inconvenient in most hospitals. Sampling for growth hormone levels every 10 to 15 minutes for 24 or 12 hours has been suggested as a way to determine if a normal circadian rhythm of growth hormone secretion is present; the facilities for such a study are generally unavailable and the actual benefit over customary secretagogue administration in diagnosis is not yet established.

Secretagogues invoked in the testing for growth hormone deficiency are given the first thing in the morning after an overnight fast. Two tests are usually performed because any normal child can fail to raise growth hormone concentration after one test in many cases. *L-Dopa* in doses of 125 mg for body weight up to 15 kg, 250 mg for weight up to 35 kg and 500 mg for body weight over 35 kg is given; samples are taken at 0, 30, 60 and 90 minutes. Nausea and vomiting are possible side effects for a few hours. *Clonidine* in a dose of 0.1 to 0.15 mg/m^2 can be given and samples obtained at the same time sequence; side effects are some hypotension and lethargy for several hours. Intravenous *arginine infusion* of 0.5 g/kg body weight up to 20 g over 20 minutes can be given with samples taken at the same time periods above; no side effects are likely. *Insulin-induced hypoglycemia* (after 0.075 to 0.1 units/kg body weight of insulin intravenously) is an effective but extremely dangerous test; the patient must be shown to have a normal fasting blood sugar just before the test, must not have a known tendency towards hypoglycemia, a patent intravenous line must be available to infuse dextrose should a hypoglycemic seizure occur, and the patient must be watched carefully by a physician during the test. If severe hypoglycemia occurs, dextrose must be administered immediately, but no more than 25% dextrose at 1 ml/kg should be infused so that blood sugar will rise, but no severe change in osmolality will occur. Glucose and growth hormone should be measured at 0, 15, 20, 30, 60, 90 minutes and cortisol at 60 and 90 minutes if this test is performed.

Growth hormone releasing factor (GHRH) is presently in use in clinical research settings, but is not commercially available. When administered in a dose of 5 to 10 μg/kg, serum growth hormone concentrations will promptly rise in normal individuals. Growth hormone deficient patients demonstrate either no rise in GH or a blunted rise; it is not always clear why one patient shows one pattern and one another.

Plasma somatomedin concentrations can be used to assist in the diagnosis of growth hormone deficiency but must be used with caution. Low values may mean malnutrition as well as growth hormone deficiency; in malnutrition growth hormone values usually rise and somatomedin values fall. In delayed puberty, values are more appropriate for bone age than chronological age and may be incorrectly interpreted as abnormally low in such a situation. The measurement of IGF-2 in addition to IGF-1 may add accuracy to the diagnosis of growth hormone deficiency, but IGF-2 determinations are not generally available. Lastly, growth hormone deficiency, or the need for growth hormone in a poorly growing child, is quite compatible with a normal somatomedin concentration. Thus, IGF-1 measurements cannot be recommended as a sole instrument for the diagnosis of growth hormone deficiency.

Treatment of Growth Hormone Deficiency

The treatment of growth hormone deficiency is presently accomplished by the use of *biosynthetic recombinant DNA-derived growth hormone*. Previously, cadaver-donated pituitary-derived growth hormone was administered, but the possibility that some batches were contaminated with the prions of Jakob-Creutzfeld disease led to the discontinuation of such therapy. Biosynthetic growth hormone is available with an N terminal methionyl group in a 192 amino acid form (given at 0.05 to 0.1 mg/kg three times per week) from Genentech or in the 191 amino acid form (given at 0.06 mg/kg three times per week) from Lilly. Previously given intramuscularly, it has been proved acceptable to inject GH subcutaneously. Recent evidence suggests that daily injections may be more effective than the classic three times per week regimen even if the total weekly dose is kept constant.

Clinical research trials have demonstrated a role for GHRH in the treatment of growth hormone deficiency: as the defect in the patient appears to be a lack of GHRH in most cases, the administration of GHRH can reverse the growth hormone deficiency in many. New methods of administering GHRH which do not require a computerized ambulatory pump are now under study. At present, no child has been treated with somatomedin.

Growth hormone presently is indicated only for growth hormone deficient patients who cannot raise growth hormone concentrations after secretagogue testing. Several studies have shown that children who are abnormally short (well below the fifth percentile), who are growing poorly (below the fifth percentile of growth velocity for age), and who have delayed bone ages (more than two standard deviations) can in about 50% of cases increase their growth rate with growth hormone therapy even though they have normal growth hormone secretion to secretagogue testing.

Children who meet these criteria are quite rare. Thus, there is a limited call for administration of growth hormone to nongrowth hormone deficient children; however, this should not suggest license to administer freely this therapy to any child below the mean for age or when parents desire their child to be taller than average. Further, there is no proved benefit for growth hormone administration in weight lifters or athletes. The theoretical or actual side effects of growth hormone administered when not indicated range from glucose intolerance to acromegalic organomegaly and even a tendency to develop slipped capital femoral epiphyses.

Psychological support is essential for the short child whether therapy is possible or not. Parents should be counseled against thinking that the fact that their child is shorter than average is a tragedy. In view of the constant bombardment by the media that leadership, friendship and indeed the company of the opposite sex requires tall stature, some boys (and rarely girls) may become severely depressed and possibly suicidal. If the parents are shorter than average and unhappy about it, they will tend to read into the child's future unpleasant experiences that they had which may not directly reflect upon their height. Children should be counseled toward sports that realistically will allow success and foster self-confidence; for example, soccer is far more appropriate than basketball. Patients who can be treated for short stature likewise will need support as they may continue to think of themselves as shorter than their peers even as the condition is resolving. Presently available data (admittedly limited) on intelligence, vocational achievement and psychosexual function suggest a variable outcome ranging from normal function to decreased function in all fields. The ultimate psychological outlook may result, to large part, from the manner in which the child was handled by family, teachers, peers and physicians during the early years after the diagnosis.

Other Endocrine Disorders

Psychosocial dwarfism may occur in one child among several other normal siblings. Abnormal parent-child interaction apparently leads to functional hypopituitarism with growth hormone deficiency on provocative testing; growth hormone secretion will quickly revert to normal after removal from the offending situation. Affected children will have a pot-bellied, immature appearance. They may drink from toilet bowls, beg for food from neighbors, forage in garbage cans in spite of apparently normal caloric intake at home. These patients may have suffered psychological abuse but may not have signs of physical abuse. When removed from their homes such children may exhibit catch-up growth in foster homes or in the hospital, but psychotherapy is needed for prolonged follow-up periods.

Maternal deprivation (perhaps a sexist term, but as the mother usually is responsible for feeding the child, often an accurate term) is the diagnosis applied to infants with poor growth rates due to parental neglect. These children may have actual caloric deprivation in addition to psychological neglect.

Hypothyroidism will decrease growth rate and retard skeletal development. Most children with congenital hypothyroidism will be diagnosed by neonatal screening procedures, but acquired hypothyroidism is still a frequent occurrence (see Chapter 7).

Cushing syndrome refers to excess glucocorticoid exposure due to endogenous or exogenous sources. Even topical preparations of glucocorticoid can retard growth and must be considered as a potential cause of decreased growth (see Chapter 5).

Pseudohypoparathyroidism presents with chubby appearance, short stature, short fourth metacarpals, round facies and mental retardation. Hypocalcemia and hyper-phosphatemia can be treated with medical therapy, but the poor growth cannot be improved by this method (see Chapter 8).

Diagnosis of Short Stature

A patient who has stature below the third percentile for height, who is growing at a rate less than the fifth percentile or is below the fifth percentile for midparental height is worthy of evaluation; a combination of two or more of these characteristics warrant increased concern. A full history and physical examination are essential for the evaluation of short stature to reveal familial influences or systemic diseases. Interfamilial interactions can be observed during the interview process to evaluate the possibility of psychosocial dwarfism. If no previous height measurements are available, a history of changes in shoe or clothing size should be of value to determine if the child is growing adequately.

Physical examination begins with the accurate measurement of height, weight, head circumference, arm span, upper to lower ratio, and vital signs. Height and height velocity are plotted on appropriate charts (see Appendix I). Height for weight ratio can be determined using charts available on the growth charts. Signs of disease or syndromes are evaluated.

If no diagnosis is obvious from history or physical, laboratory evaluation is performed. A screening chemistry panel for liver and kidney function, a bicarbonate and electrolyte determination to evaluate the possibility of renal tubular acidosis or a metabolic acidosis syndrome, a carotene determination for an index of fat absorption, a complete blood count, a sedimentation rate, and a urinalysis including microscopic exam may indicate a problem not obvious from the physical examination. A free thyroxine determination or a thyroid test with an indication of the level of binding protein also is obtained. A somatomedin concentration may be falsely low due to factors listed before, but if the somatomedin is normal, classic growth hormone deficiency is far less likely. A urinary-free cortisol or urinary 17-OHCS excretion determination is obtained if obesity complicates short stature. A prolactin concentration, if elevated, will suggest hypothalamic deficiency. A bone age determination will not lead to a diagnosis (although it may support potential diagnoses), but it will indicate the amount of remaining growth left. If neurologic symptoms are noted or if a central nervous system tumor is in the differential diagnosis, a radiologic evaluation of the pituitary-hypothalamic area is in order; in the past, a lateral x-ray of the skull was performed, but presently a computerized tomographic (CT) with contrast or a magnetic resonance imaging study (MRI) scan is considered appropriate. If a CT scan is performed, it is essential that thin cuts are taken through the hypothalamic-pituitary area so that a small tumor or congenital abnormality is not missed.

Growth hormone testing is performed if no other diagnosis is apparent from the above evaluation. As mentioned above, the diagnosis of classic growth hormone deficiency is relatively straightforward, but the emergence of other, more subtle conditions where growth hormone treatment may be helpful has confused the situation. Growth hormone is not generally available except for growth hormone deficiency, and the decision to treat nonclassical patients at present should rest with a pediatric endocrinologist. At present the companies producing growth hormone will only allow it to be prescribed by specialists dealing with pediatric endocrinology, but the time will likely come when such treatment is more easily available to physicians less experienced with its use; abuses of biosynthetic GH can be expected to follow the pattern of those found with natural pituitary derived growth hormone in the past. Treatment with growth hormone has been detailed above.

Tall Stature

Nonendocrine Causes of Tall Stature

Constitutional tall stature is the other side of the coin from constitutional short stature. Patients are taller than average, have a moderately advanced bone age but a height velocity appropriate for bone age, and have no sign of the disorders described below. Often the patients are obese, as obesity will advance bone age and physiologic development. Puberty will be early in children with constitutional tall stature so that final height will not be out of normal range, although height during childhood was greater than normal.

Genetic tall stature occurs in a family with one or, more often, two parents taller than the normal adult range. The child will be born at a normal length and weight but, because of high normal growth rate, will reach a height more than two standard deviations above the mean without appreciable advance in bone age. Thus, their height as adults will be taller than average.

In today's society, girls more often will be concerned about being taller than average than will boys; often fears are intensified by parental concerns about tall stature and effects on social development. Treatment with high-dose estrogens can effectively slow longitudinal growth while advancing puberty, causing a rapid increase in bone age and thereby limiting adult height in girls. Because of theoretic risks of high-dose estrogen therapy, such as thrombotic effects, the development of ovarian cysts and, in fact, future menstrual disorders, therapy is not to be undertaken without a careful description of the possible side effects. Further, the child must be included in discussions concerning her adult height. In rare circumstances, a girl with a predicted height of more than 6 feet, who is 10 to 12 years of age with a bone age no older than 10 to 11 years, may hope to realize a decrease in her final height of up to 2 inches with the use of estrogen therapy.

Boys concerned about too great a final height are rare, but testosterone therapy can be used to precipitate pubertal development and limit final height.

Cerebral gigantism is recognized by the prominent forehead and sharp chin, high-arched palate, hypertelorism and often developmental delay with no evidence of growth hormone excess. Rapid growth is most characteristic of infancy and height velocity decreases by mid-childhood.

Marfan syndrome, or *arachnodactyly*, includes tall stature (with arm span exceeding height and a very low upper to lower segment ratio), long, thin fingers and toes, hyperextensibility of the joints, subluxation of the lens, and aortic dilation.

Homocystinuria causes a phenotype somewhat reminiscent of Marfan syndrome. Mental retardation is characteristic of homocystinuria as is increased excretion of homocystine in the urine.

Beckwith-Wiedemann syndrome leads to very large newborn length and weight, omphalocele and macroglossia. Life threatening hypoglycemia occurs because of hyperinsulinism due to pancreatic hyperplasia. In addition, there will be fetal adrenocortical cytomegaly and large kidneys with medullary dysplasia. Body size remains large throughout childhood.

Syndromes with extra Y chromosomes such as *47XYY* or *48XYYY* lead to tall stature in childhood and adult life without any evidence of increased growth hormone. *Klinefelter's syndrome (47XXY)* may be associated with tall stature.

Endocrine Etiologies of Tall Stature

Pituitary gigantism is due to a growth hormone secreting adenoma in childhood; acromegaly is the occurrence of the same type of tumor in an adult. Because the epiphyses are not closed in an affected child, height velocity is increased although the coarse features of an acromegalic appearance also may be noted. Organomegaly may occur and glucose intolerance or frank diabetes may result. Elevated fasting growth hormone concentrations or somatomedin levels confirm the diagnosis.

Precocious puberty of any etiology increases growth in childhood, but early epiphyseal closure and short adult stature will result.

Thyrotoxicosis increases height velocity and skeletal age advancement.

Infants of diabetic mothers are large at birth but postnatal growth is normal. Fetal hyperinsulinism is the stimulus for the excessive fetal growth; neonatal hypoglycemia can be a serious complication, as the high maternal glucose concentration that led to the fetal hyperinsulinism is removed at the time of birth.

Children with *β-cell adenomas* may have continued rapid growth during their hyperinsulinemic state, but their hypoglycemia will most likely of be the clinical condition that brings them to diagnosis.

Diagnosis and Treatment of Tall Stature

Generally, the historical and physical manifestations of precocious puberty, hyperthyroidism, Marfan syndrome, homocystinuria, cerebral gigantism and insulin excess are evident during the history and physical exam so that these causes of tall stature can be investigated directly. Initial differentiation between pituitary gigantism and constitutional or genetic tall stature may be more difficult. This is one case in which a somatomedin concentration can be quite useful if it is remembered that during puberty somatomedin concentrations rise as high as the concentrations that would be encountered in a younger child with bona fide pituitary gigantism. Basal growth hormone concentration also should be elevated in pituitary gigantism when compared with the low concentrations seen in normal subjects. Pituitary giants also respond with growth hormone secretion to agents that normally do not stimulate growth hormone secretion, agents such as glucose infusion (normally glucose suppresses growth hormone), gonadotropin releasing hormone (GnRH) and thyrotropin releasing factor (TRF) (both of which normally have no effect on growth hormone secretion).

Patients with tumors stimulating their growth are amenable to surgical removal of their tumor. Those with hyperthyroidism and precocious puberty are amenable to therapy as described in the chapters that consider these disorders. Pituitary gigantism is treated by transphenoidal microadenomectomy if the technical expertise is available.

Suggested Readings

Aynsley-Green A, Zachmann M, Prader A: Interrelation of the therapeutic effects of growth hormone and testosterone on growth in hypopituitarism. J Pediatr 1976;89:992

Bercu BB: Growth hormone treatment and the short child: to treat or not to treat? J Pedatr 1987;110:991

Clarren SK, Smithy DW: The fetal alcohol syndrome.   N Engl J Med 1978;298:1063

Conte FA, Grumbach MM: Epidemiological aspects of estrogen use: estrogen use in children and adolescents: A survey.   Pediatrics 1978;62:1091

Dean HJ, Bishop A, Winter JSD: Growth hormone deficiency in patients with histiocytosis. J Pediatr 1986;109:615

Greulich WW, Pyle SII: Radiographic Atlas of Skeletal Development of the Hand and Wrist,   2nd ed.   Stanford, CA: Stanford University Press, 1959

Himes JH, Roche AF, Thissen D: Parent   specific adjustments for assessment of recumbent length and stature. vol 13, Monographs in Paediatrics, Karger, 1981

Lovinger RD, Kaplan SL, Grumbach MM: Congenital hypopituitarism associated with neonatal hypoglycemia and microphallus; Four cases secondary to hypothalamic hormone deficiencies.   J Pediatr 1975; 87:1171

Mazur T, Clopper RR: Hypopituitarism: Review of behavioral data. In: Current Concepts in Pediatric Endocrinology. Styne DM, Brook CGD (editors). New York: Elsevier, 1987, p 184

Plotnich JP, Lee PA, Migeon CJ, Kowarski AA, et al: Comparison of physiological test of growth hormone function in children with short stature. J Clin Endocrinol Metab 1979;48:811

Rosenfeld RG, Wilson DW, Lee PDK, Hintz RL: Insulin-like growth factors I and II in evaluation of growth retardation.   J Pedaitr 1986;109:317

Rosenfeld RG, Hintz RL, Johanson A, et al: Methionyl human growth hormone and oxandrolone in Turner syndrome; Preliminary results of a prospective randomized trial.   J Pediatr 1986;109:936

Raiti S, Tolman RA: Human Growth Hormone. New York: Plenum Medical Book Company, 1986

Raiti SR, Moore WV, Van Vliet G, Kaplan SL: Growth-stimulating effects of human growth hormone therapy in patients with Turner syndrome.   J Pediatr 1986;109:944

Richards GE, Wara WM, Grumbach MM, et al: Delayed onset of hypopituitarism; sequelae of therapeutic irradiation of central nervous system and middle ear tumors.   J Pediatr 1976;89:553

Roche AF, Himes, JH: Incremental growth charts.   Am J Clin Nutr 1980;333:2041

Roche AF, Wainer H, Thissen D: The RWT method for the prediction of adult stature.   Pediatrics 197;56:1026

Ross JL, Long LM, Skerda M, et al: Effect of low dose of estradiol on 67-month growth rates and predicted height in patients with Turner syndrome.   J Pediatr 1986;109:905

Rudman D, Davis GT, Priest JH, et al: Prevalence of growth hormone deficiency in children with cleft lip or palate.   J Pediatr 1978;98:378

Styne DM: Growth. In: Basic and Clinical Endocrinology. Greenspan F, Forsham P (editors); San Mateo, CA: Lange Medical Pub, 1986 p 107

Tanner JM, Davies PSW: Clinical longitudinal standard for height and height velocity for North American Children.   J Pediatr 1985: 107:317

Tanner JM, Whitehouse RH, Hughes PCR, Carter BS: Relative importance of growth hormone and sex steroids for the growth of puberty of trunk length, limb length and muscle width in growth hormone deficient children.   J Pediatr 1976;89:1000

Van Vliet G, et al: Growth hormone can increase growth rate in short normal children: evaluation of the somatomedin-C generation test in the assessment of children with short stature.   N Engl J Med 1983;309:1016

Zachmann M, Praeder A, Sobel EH, et al: Pubertal growth in patients with androgen insensitivity: indirect evidence for the importance of estrogen in pubertal growth of girls.   J Pediatr 1986;108:694

APPENDIX 1

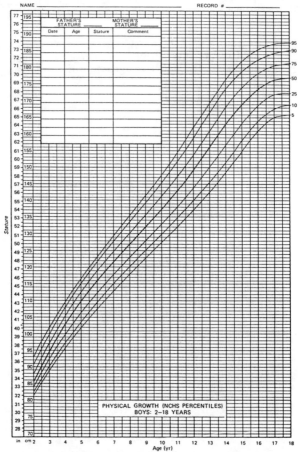

Growth chart for boys in the USA. (redrawn by Appleton & Lange and reprinted with permission of Ross Laboratories, Columbus, OH 43216 and Appleton & Lange, San Mateo, CA. Copyright Ross Laboratories. Source of data: 1976 study of the National Center for Health Statistics [NICHS; Hyattsville, MD]; Hamill PVV et al; Physical growth: National Center for Health Statistics percentiles Am J Clin Nutr 1979;32:607.)

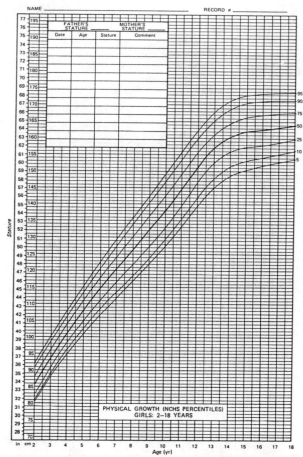

Growth chart for girls in the USA. (redrawn by Appleton & Lange and reprinted with permission of Ross Laboratories, Columbus, OH 43216 and Appleton & Lange, San Mateo, CA. Copyright Ross Laboratories. Source of data: 1976 study of the National Center for Health Statistics [NICHS; Hyattsville, MD]; Hamill PVV et al; Physical growth: National Center for Health Statistics percentiles. Am J Clin Nutr 1979;32:607.)

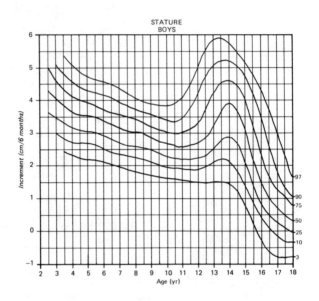

Incremental growth charts for boys. Height velocity measured over a period of at least 6 months can be compared with the percentiles on the right axis of the charts. (Redrawn by Appleton & Lange with permission of Ross Laboratories, Columbus OH 43216 and Appleton & Lange, San Mateo, CA. Copyright Ross Laboratories. Source of data: Longitudinal studies of the Fels Research Laboratories [Yellow Springs, OH]; Roche AF, Himes JH: Incremental growth charts. Am J Clin Nutr 1980;33:204.)

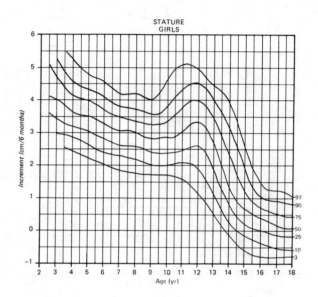

Incremental growth charts for girls. Height velocity measured over a period of at least 6 months can be compared with the percentiles on the right axis of the charts. (Redrawn by Appleton & Lange with permission of Ross Laboratories, Columbus OH 43216 and Appleton & Lange, San Mateo, CA. Copyright Ross Laboratories. Source of data: Longitudinal studies of the Fels Research Laboratories [Yellow Springs, OH]; Roche AF, Himes JH: Incremental growth charts. Am J Clin Nutr 1980;33:204.)

PARENT SPECIFIC ADJUSTMENTS (CM) FOR STATURE OF BOYS

Age (yr)	Stature (cm)	Mid Parental Stature (cm)																	
		150	152	154	156	158	160	162	164	166	168	170	172	174	176	178	180	182	184
3	86.0– 87.9	7	6	5	5	4	3	2	1	1	0	-1	-2	-3	-3	-4	-5	-6	-7
	88.0– 97.9	8	7	6	5	4	4	3	2	1	0	-1	-1	-2	-3	-4	-5	-5	-6
	98.0–106.9	8	8	7	6	5	4	4	3	2	1	0	0	1	-2	-3	-4	-4	-5
4	90.0– 93.9	7	6	5	4	4	3	2	1	0	-1	-1	-2	-3	-4	-5	-5	-6	-7
	94.0–103.9	8	7	6	5	4	3	3	2	1	0	-1	-1	-2	-3	-4	-5	-6	-6
	104.0–112.9	8	8	7	6	5	4	3	3	2	1	0	-1	-1	-2	-3	-4	-5	-6
5	96.0–103.9	8	7	6	5	4	3	2	1	0	0	-1	-2	-3	-4	-5	-6	-7	-8
	104.0–113.9	9	8	7	6	5	4	3	2	1	0	0	-1	-2	-3	-4	-5	-6	-7
	114.0–122.9	9	9	8	7	6	5	4	3	2	1	0	0	-1	-2	-3	-4	-5	-6
6	102.0–111.9	8	7	7	6	5	4	3	2	1	0	-1	-2	-3	-4	-5	-6	-7	-8·
	112.0–121.9	9	8	7	7	6	5	4	3	2	1	0	-1	-2	-3	-4	-5	-6	-7
	122.0–130.9	10	9	8	7	6	6	5	4	3	2	1	0	-1	-2	-3	-4	-5	-6
7	108.0–117.9	9	8	7	6	5	4	3	2	1	0	-1	-2	-4	-5	-6	-7	-8	-9
	118.0–127.9	10	9	8	7	6	5	4	3	2	1	0	-1	-2	-4	-5	-6	-7	-8
	128.0–136.9	12	10	9	8	7	6	5	4	3	2	1	0	-1	-2	-4	-5	-6	-7
8	114.0–115.9	10	9	8	6	5	4	3	2	1	-1	-2	-3	-4	-5	-6	-8	-9	-10
	116.0–125.9	11	9	8	7	6	5	4	2	1	0	-1	-2	-3	-5	-6	-7	-8	-9
	126.0–135.9	12	10	9	8	7	6	5	3	2	1	0	-1	-2	-4	-5	-6	-7	-8
	136.0–144.9	13	12	10	9	8	7	6	5	3	2	1	0	-1	-2	-4	-5	-6	-7
9	120.0–121.9	11	9	8	7	6	4	3	2	1	0	-2	-3	-4	-5	-7	-8	-9	-10
	122.0–131.9	11	10	9	8	6	5	4	3	1	0	-1	-2	-3	-5	-6	-7	-8	-10
	132.0–141.9	12	11	10	9	7	6	5	4	2	1	0	-1	-2	-4	-5	-6	-7	-9
	142.0–150.9	13	12	11	10	8	7	6	5	4	2	1	0	-1	-3	-4	-5	-6	-7
10	124.0–127.9	11	10	9	7	6	5	3	2	1	-1	-2	-3	-5	-6	-7	-9	-10	-11
	128.0–137.9	12	11	10	8	7	6	4	3	2	0	-1	-2	-4	-5	-6	-8	-9	-10
	138.0–147.9	13	12	11	9	8	7	5	4	3	1	0	-1	-3	-4	-5	-7	-8	-9
	148.0–158.9	14	13	12	11	9	8	7	5	4	3	1	0	-1	-3	-4	-5	-7	-8
11	128.0–133.9	12	10	9	8	6	5	4	2	1	0	-2	-3	-5	-6	-7	-9	-10	-11
	134.0–143.9	12	11	10	8	7	6	4	3	2	0	-1	-2	-4	-5	-6	-8	-9	-10
	144.0–153.9	14	12	11	10	8	7	5	4	3	1	0	-1	-3	-4	-5	-7	-8	-9
	154.0–162.9	15	13	12	11	9	8	7	5	4	3	1	0	-2	-3	-4	-6	-7	-8
12	132.0–141.9	12	10	9	8	6	5	4	2	1	0	-2	-3	-4	-6	-7	-8	-10	-11
	142.0–151.9	13	11	10	9	7	6	5	3	2	1	-1	-2	-3	-5	-6	-7	-9	-10
	152.0–161.9	13	12	11	9	8	7	5	4	3	1	0	-1	-2	-4	-5	-6	-8	-9
	162.0–170.9	14	13	12	10	9	8	6	5	4	2	1	0	-2	-3	-4	-6	-7	-8
13	136.0–139.9	12	10	9	8	6	5	4	2	1	-1	-2	-3	-5	-6	-7	-9	-10	-12
	140.0–149.9	12	11	10	8	7	6	4	3	1	0	-1	-3	-4	-6	-7	-8	-10	-11
	150.0–159.9	13	12	10	9	8	6	5	4	2	1	-1	-2	-3	-5	-6	-7	-9	-10
	160.0–169.9	14	13	11	10	8	7	6	4	3	2	0	-1	-3	-4	-5	-7	-8	-9
	170.0–178.9	15	13	12	11	9	8	6	5	4	2	1	0	-2	-3	-5	-6	-7	-9
14	142.0–145.9	13	11	10	8	7	5	4	2	1	-1	-2	-4	-5	-7	-8	-10	-11	-13
	146.0–155.9	14	12	11	9	8	6	5	3	1	0	-2	-3	-5	-6	-8	-9	-11	-12
	156.0–165.9	15	13	11	10	8	7	5	4	2	1	-1	-2	-4	-5	-7	-8	-9	-11
	166.0–175.9	15	14	12	11	9	8	6	5	3	2	0	-1	-3	-4	-6	-7	-9	-11
	176.0–184.9	16	15	13	12	10	9	7	6	4	3	1	-1	-2	-4	-5	-7	-8	-10
15	148.0–151.9	14	13	11	9	7	6	4	2	0	-1	-3	-5	-7	-8	-10	-12	-14	-15
	152.0–161.9	15	14	12	10	8	7	5	3	1	0	-2	-4	-6	-7	-9	-11	-13	-14
	162.0–171.9	17	15	13	11	10	8	6	4	3	1	-1	-3	-4	-6	-8	-10	-11	-13
	172.0–181.9	18	16	14	13	11	9	7	6	4	2	0	-1	-3	-5	-7	-8	-10	-12
	182.0–192.9	19	17	16	14	12	10	9	7	5	3	2	0	-2	-4	-6	-7	-9	-11
16	156.0–163.9	17	15	13	11	9	7	5	3	1	-1	-3	-5	-7	-9	-11	-13	-16	-18
	164.0–173.9	19	17	15	13	10	8	6	4	2	0	-2	-4	-6	-8	-10	-12	-14	-16
	174.0–183.9	21	19	17	15	12	10	8	6	4	2	0	-2	-4	-6	-8	-10	-12	-14
	184.0–192.9	23	21	19	17	14	12	10	8	6	4	2	0	-2	-4	-6	-8	-10	-12
17	162.0–165.9	17	15	13	11	9	7	4	2	0	-2	-4	-7	-9	-11	-13	-15	-17	-20
	166.0–175.9	20	17	15	13	11	9	6	4	2	0	-2	-4	-7	-9	-11	-13	-15	-18
	176.0–185.9	22	20	18	16	13	11	9	7	5	3	0	-2	-4	-6	-8	-11	-13	-15
	186.0–194.9	25	23	20	18	16	14	12	9	7	5	3	1	-1	-4	-6	-8	-10	-12
18	160.0–165.9	18	16	13	11	9	6	4	2	0	-3	-5	-7	-10	-12	-14	-17	-19	-21
	166.0–175.9	20	18	16	13	11	9	7	4	2	0	-3	-5	-7	-10	-12	-14	-17	-19
	176.0–185.9	23	21	19	16	14	12	9	7	5	3	0	-2	-4	-7	-9	-11	-14	-16
	186.0–194.9	26	24	22	19	17	15	12	10	8	6	3	1	-1	-4	-6	-8	-11	-13

Reprinted, with permission, from Styne DM: Growth. in: Basic and Clinical Endocrinology. Greenspan F, Forsham P (editors). San Mateo, CA: Lange Medical Publishers, 1986; p 112.

PARENT SPECIFIC ADJUSTMENTS (CM) FOR STATURE OF BOYS

Age (yr)	Stature (cm)	Mid Parental Stature (cm)																	
		150	152	154	156	158	160	162	164	166	168	170	172	174	176	178	180	182	184
3	82.0– 83.9	6	5	4	4	3	2	1	1	0	-1	-1	-2	-3	-3	-4	-5	-6	-6
	84.0– 93.9	6	6	5	4	3	3	2	1	1	0	-1	-1	-2	-3	-4	-4	-5	-6
	94.0–102.9	7	7	6	5	4	4	3	2	2	1	0	-1	-1	-2	-3	-3	-4	-5
4	92.0– 93.9	6	6	5	4	3	3	2	1	0	0	-1	-2	-3	-3	-4	-5	-6	-7
	94.0–103.9	7	6	6	5	4	3	2	2	1	0	-1	-1	-2	-3	-4	-4	-5	-6
	104.0–112.9	8	7	7	6	5	4	3	3	2	1	0	0	-1	-2	-3	-3	-4	-5
5	100.0–101.9	8	7	6	5	4	3	2	1	1	0	-1	-2	-3	-4	-5	-5	-6	-7
	102.0–111.9	8	7	6	6	5	4	3	2	1	0	-1	-1	-2	-3	-4	-5	-6	-7
	112.0–120.9	9	8	7	7	6	5	4	3	2	1	1	0	-1	-2	-3	-4	-5	-6
6	106.0–109.9	9	8	7	6	5	4	3	2	1	0	-1	-2	-3	-4	-5	-6	-7	-8
	110.0–119.9	9	9	8	7	6	5	4	3	2	1	0	-1	-2	-3	-4	-5	-6	-7
	120.0–128.9	11	10	9	8	7	6	5	4	3	2	1	0	-1	-2	-3	-4	-5	-6
7	112.0–117.9	9	8	7	6	5	4	3	2	1	0	-1	-2	-3	-4	-5	-6	-7	-8
	118.0–127.9	10	9	8	7	6	5	4	3	2	1	0	-1	-2	-3	-4	-5	-6	-7
	128.0–136.9	11	10	9	8	7	6	5	4	3	2	1	0	-1	-2	-3	-4	-5	-6
8	116.0–123.9	9	8	7	6	5	4	3	2	1	0	-1	-2	-3	-4	-5	-6	-8	-9
	124.0–133.9	10	9	8	7	6	5	4	3	2	1	0	-1	-2	-3	-4	-5	-7	-8
	134.0–142.9	11	10	9	8	7	6	5	4	3	2	1	0	-1	-2	-3	-4	-6	-7
9	122.0–131.9	10	9	8	7	6	5	3	2	1	0	-1	-2	-3	-4	-5	-6	-7	-9
	132.0–141.9	11	10	9	8	7	6	4	3	2	1	0	-1	-2	-3	-4	-5	-7	-8
	142.0–150.9	12	11	10	9	8	6	5	4	3	2	1	0	-1	-2	-3	-4	-6	-7
10	126.0–127.9	10	9	7	6	5	4	3	2	1	0	-1	-2	-3	-5	-6	-7	-8	-9
	128.0–137.9	10	9	8	7	6	5	4	2	1	0	-1	-2	-3	-4	-5	-6	-7	-8
	138.0–147.9	11	10	9	8	6	5	4	3	2	1	0	-1	-2	-3	-4	-5	-7	-8
	148.0–156.9	12	10	9	8	7	6	5	4	3	2	1	0	-1	-3	-4	-5	-6	-7
11	130.0–133.9	10	9	8	6	5	4	3	2	1	0	-1	-2	-3	-4	-6	-7	-8	-9
	134.0–143.9	10	9	8	7	6	5	4	3	1	0	-1	-2	-3	-4	-5	-6	-7	-8
	144.0–153.9	11	10	9	7	6	5	4	3	2	1	0	-1	-2	-3	-5	-6	-7	-8
	154.0–162.9	11	10	9	8	7	6	5	4	3	1	0	-1	-2	-3	-4	-5	-6	-7
12	134.0–139.9	10	9	8	7	6	5	3	2	1	0	-1	-3	-4	-5	-6	-7	-8	-10
	140.0–149.9	11	10	9	7	6	5	4	3	2	0	-1	-2	-3	-4	-6	-7	-8	-9
	150.0–159.9	12	10	9	8	7	6	5	3	2	1	0	-1	-3	-4	-5	-6	-7	-8
	160.0–168.9	12	11	10	9	8	6	5	4	3	2	0	-1	-2	-3	-4	-5	-7	-8
13	140.0–145.9	10	9	8	7	6	4	3	2	1	0	-1	-3	-4	-5	-6	-7	-8	-10
	146.0–155.9	11	10	9	7	6	5	4	3	2	0	-1	-2	-3	-4	-6	-7	-8	-9
	156.0–165.9	12	10	9	8	7	6	5	3	2	1	0	-1	-3	-4	-5	-6	-7	-8
	166.0–174.9	12	11	10	9	8	6	5	4	3	2	1	-1	-2	-3	-4	-5	-7	-8
14	146.0–149.9	10	9	8	6	5	4	3	2	1	0	-1	-3	-4	-5	-6	-7	-8	-9
	150.0–159.9	11	9	8	7	6	5	4	3	1	0	-1	-2	-3	-4	-5	-7	-8	-9
	160.0–169.9	11	10	9	8	7	6	5	3	2	1	0	-1	-2	-3	-5	-6	-7	-8
	170.0–178.9	12	11	10	9	8	6	5	4	3	2	1	0	-2	-3	-4	-5	-6	-7
15	146.0–151.9	10	9	8	7	5	4	3	2	1	-1	-2	-3	-4	-5	-6	-8	-9	-10
	152.0–161.9	11	10	9	7	6	5	4	3	1	0	-1	-2	-3	-4	-6	-7	-8	-9
	162.0–171.9	12	11	10	8	7	6	5	4	2	1	0	-1	-2	-4	-5	-6	-7	-8
	172.0–180.9	13	12	11	9	8	7	6	5	3	2	1	0	-1	-3	-4	-5	-6	-7
16	146.0–151.9	11	10	8	7	6	5	3	2	1	-1	-2	-3	-4	-6	-7	-8	-10	-11
	152.0–161.9	12	10	9	8	7	5	4	3	2	0	-1	-2	-4	-5	-6	-7	-9	-10
	162.0–171.9	13	12	10	9	8	6	5	4	3	1	0	-1	-3	-4	-5	-6	-8	-9
	172.0–180.9	14	13	11	10	9	7	6	5	4	2	1	0	-2	-3	-4	-5	-7	-8
17	148.0–153.9	11	10	9	7	6	5	3	2	1	0	-2	-3	-4	-6	-7	-8	-10	-11
	154.0–163.9	12	11	10	8	7	6	4	3	2	0	-1	-2	-4	-5	-6	-8	-9	-10
	164.0–173.9	13	12	11	9	8	7	5	4	3	1	0	-1	-3	-4	-5	-6	-8	-9
	174.0–182.9	14	13	12	10	9	8	6	5	4	2	1	0	-1	-3	-4	-5	-7	-8
18	148.0–149.9	10	9	8	7	5	4	3	2	1	-1	-2	-3	-4	-6	-7	-8	-9	-10
	150.0–159.9	11	10	8	7	6	5	4	2	1	0	-1	-3	-4	-5	-6	-7	-9	-10
	160.0–169.9	12	11	9	8	7	6	4	3	2	1	0	-2	-3	-4	-5	-6	-8	-9
	170.0–178.9	13	11	10	9	8	7	5	4	3	2	1	-1	-2	-3	-4	-5	-7	-8

Reprinted, with permission, from Styne DM: Growth. in: Basic and Clincal Endocrinology. Greenspan F, Forsham P (editors). San Mateo, CA: Lange Medical Publishers, 1986; p 113.

THE RWT METHOD FOR PREDICTING ADULT STATURE

(From Roche AF, Wainer H, Thissen D: The RWT method for the prediction of adult stature. Pediatrics 1975;56:1026, as modified in Styne DM: Growth Disorders. in; Fitzgerald PA (editor) <u>Handbook of Clinical Endocrinology</u> Greenbrae, CA: Jones Medical Publication. 1986 p 99).

The RWT method predicts the height of an individual at 18 years of age; after this age the average total increase in stature is 0.6 cm for girls and 0.8 cm for boys.

Recumbent length is measured in cm (add 1.25 cm to the standing height, without shoes, if that is available). Weight is measured in kg. The *midparental height* is calculated by adding the standing height of each parent in cm (without shoes) and dividing by two; if the parents' heights are unknown, in the USA a height of 174.5 cm can be substituted for the father's height or 162 cm for the mother's height. The skeletal age is determined from an x-ray of the left wrist and hand and comparing it to the Greulich and Pyle atlas.

A prediction is made by:

1. Recording the child's data as noted below.
2. Finding the multipliers from the charts on the next two pages; make sure the positive and negative signs are retained for the calculations.
3. Multiply the data by the multipliers taking note of the positive or negative sign.
4. Add the products to the adjustment factor taking note of the sign of the factor: the result is a prediction of the height at 18 years of age.

DATA	MULTIPLIERS		PRODUCTS
Recumbent length (cm)	x_____	=	_____
Weight (kg)	x_____	=	_____
Midparental stature (cm)	x_____	=	_____
Skeletal age (years)	x_____	=	_____
Adjustment factor for age		=	+ /-_____
Predicted height at age 18 years (cm)		=	_____

TABLES OF MULTIPLIERS FOR PREDICTION OF ADULT STATURE IN BOYS BY THE RWT METHOD

Age Yrs	Mos	Recumbent length	Weight	Midparental stature	Skeletal age	Adjustment factor
1	0	0.966	0.199	0.606	−0.673	1.632
1	3	1.032	0.086	0.580	−0.417	−1.841
1	6	1.086	−0.016	0.559	−0.205	−4.892
1	9	1.130	−0.106	0.540	−0.033	−7.528
2	0	1.163	−0.186	0.523	0.104	−9.764
2	3	1.189	−0.256	0.509	0.211	−11.618
2	6	1.207	−0.316	0.496	0.291	−13.114
2	9	1.219	−0.369	0.485	0.349	−14.278
3	0	1.227	−0.413	0.475	0.388	−15.139
3	3	1.230	−0.450	0.466	0.410	−15.729
3	6	1.229	−0.481	0.458	0.419	−16.081
3	9	1.226	−0.505	0.451	0.417	−16.228
4	0	1.221	−0.523	0.444	0.405	−16.201
4	3	1.214	−0.537	0.437	0.387	−16.034
4	6	1.206	−0.546	0.431	0.363	−15.758
4	9	1.197	−0.550	0.424	0.335	−15.400
5	0	1.188	−0.551	0.418	0.303	−14.990
5	3	1.179	−0.548	0.412	0.269	−14.551
5	6	1.169	−0.543	0.406	0.234	−14.106
5	9	1.160	−0.535	0.400	0.198	−13.672
6	0	1.152	−0.524	0.394	0.161	−13.267
6	3	1.143	−0.512	0.389	0.123	−12.901
6	6	1;135	−0.499	0.383	0.085	−12.583
6	9	1.127	−0.484	0.378	0.046	−12.318
7	0	1.120	−0.468	0.373	0.006	−12.107
7	3	1.113	−0.451	0.369	−0.034	−11.948
7	6	1.106	−0.434	0.365	−0.077	−11.834
7	9	1.100	−0.417	0.361	−0.121	−11.756
8	0	1.093	−0.400	0.358	−0.167	−11.701
8	3	1.086	−0.382	0.356	−0.217	−11.652
8	6	1.079	−0.365	0.354	−0.270	−11.592
8	9	1.071	−0.349	0.353	−0.327	−11.498
9	0	1.063	−0.333	0.353	−0.389	−11.349
9	3	1.054	−0.317	0.353	−0.455	−11.118
9	6	1.044	−0.303	0.355	−0.527	−10.779
9	9	1.033	−0.289	0.357	−0.605	−10.306
10	0	1.021	−0.276	0.360	−0.690	−9.671
10	3	1.008	−0.263	).363	−0.781	−8.848
10	6	0.993	−0.252	0.368	−0.878	−7.812
10	9	0.977	−0.241	0.373	−0.983	−6.540
11	0	0.960	−0.231	0.378	−1.094	−5.010
11	3	0.942	−0.222	0.384	−1.211	−3.206
11	6	0.923	−0.213	0.390	−1.335	−1.113
11	9	0.902	−0.206	0.397	−1.464	1.273
12	0	0.881	−0.198	0.403	−1.597	3.958
12	3	0.859	−0.191	0.409	−1.735	6.931
12	6	0.837	−0.184	0.414	−1.875	10.181
12	9	0.815	−0.177	0.418	−2.015	13.684
13	0	0.794	−0.170	0.421	−2.156	17.405
13	3	0.773	−0.163	0.422	−2.294	21.297
13	6	0.755	−0.155	0.422	−2.427	25.304
13	9	0.738	−0.146	0.418	−2.553	29.349
14	0	0.724	−0.136	0.412	−2.668	33.345
14	3	0.714	−0.125	0.401	−2.771	37.183
14	6	0.709	−0.112	0.387	−2.856	40.738
14	9	0.709	−0.098	0.367	−2.922	43.869
15	0	0.717	−0.081	0.342	−2.962	46.403
15	3	0.732	−0.062	0.310	−2.973	48.154
15	6	0.756	−0.040	0.271	−2.949	48.898
15	9	0.792	−0.015	0.223	−2.885	48.402
16	0	0.839	−0.014	0.167	−2.776	46.391

TABLES OF MULTIPLIERS FOR PREDICTION OF ADULT STATURE IN GIRLS BY THE RWT METHOD

Age Yrs	Mos	Recumbent length	Weight	Midparental stature	Skeletal age	Adjustment factor
1	0	1.087	−0.271	0.386	0.434	21.729
1	3	1.112	−0.369	0.367	0.094	20.684
1	6	1.134	−0.455	0.349	−0.172	19.957
1	9	1.153	−0.530	0.332	−0.374	19.463
2	0	1.170	−0.594	0.316	−0.523	19.131
2	3	1.183	−0.648	0.301	−0.625	18.905
2	6	1.195	−0.693	0.287	−0.690	18.740
2	9	1.204	−0.729	0.274	−0.725	18.604
3	0	1.210	−0.757	0.262	−0.736	18.474
3	3	1.215	−0.777	0.251	−0.729	18.337
3	6	1.217	−0.791	0.241	−0.711	18.187
3	9	1.217	−0.798	0.232	−0.684	18.024
4	0	1.215	−0.800	0.224	−0.655	17.855
4	3	1.212	−0.797	0.217	−0.626	17.691
4	6	1.206	−0.789	0.210	−0.600	17.548
4	9	1.199	−0.777	0.205	−0.582	17.444
5	0	1.190	−0.761	0.200	−0.571	17.398
5	3	1.180	−0.742	0.197	−0.572	17.431
5	6	1.168	−0.721	0.193	−0.584	17.567
5	9	1.155	−0.697	0.191	−0.609	17.826
6	0	1.140	−0.671	0.190	−0.647	18.229
6	3	1.124	−0.644	0.189	−0.700	18.796
6	6	1.107	−0.616	0.188	−0.766	19.544
6	9	1.089	−0.587	0.189	−0.845	20.489
7	0	1.069	−0.557	0.189	−0.938	21.642
7	3	1.049	−0.527	0.191	−1.043	23.011
7	6	1.028	−0.498	0.192	−1.158	24.602
7	9	1.006	−0.468	0.194	−1.284	26.416
8	0	0.938	−0.439	0.196	−1.418	28.448
8	3	0.960	−0.411	0.199	−1.558	30.690
8	6	0.937	−0.384	0.202	−1.704	33.129
8	9	0.914	−0.359	0.204	−1.853	35.747
9	0	0.891	−0.334	0.207	−2.003	38.520
9	3	0.868	−0.311	0.210	−2.154	41.421
9	6	0.845	−0.289	0.212	−2.301	44.415
9	9	0.824	−0.269	0.214	−2.444	47.464
10	0	0.803	−0.250	0.216	−2.581	50.525
10	3	0.783	−0.233	0.217	−2.710	53.548
10	6	0.766	−0.217	0.217	−2.829	56.481
10	9	0.749	−0.203	0.217	−2.936	59.267
11	0	0.736	−0.190	0.216	−3.029	61.841
11	3	0.724	−0.179	0.214	−3.108	84.136
11	6	0.716	−0.169	0.211	−3.171	66.093
11	9	0.711	−0.159	0.206	−3.217	67.627
12	0	0.710	−0.151	0.201	−3.245	68.670
12	3	0.713	−0.143	0.193	−3.254	69.140
12	6	0.720	−0.136	0.184	−3.244	68.966
12	9	0.733	−0.129	0.173	−3.214	68.061
13	0	0.752	−0.121	0.160	−3.166	66.339
13	3	0.777	−0.113	0.144	−3.100	63.728
13	6	0.810	−0.105	0.127	−3.015	60.150
13	9	0.850	−0.085	0.106	−2.915	55.522
14	0	0.898	−0.083	0.083	−2.800	49.781

Chapter 2

Sexual Differentiation

SEXUAL DIFFERENTIATION

The appearance of ambiguous genitalia in the newborn must be considered a emergency. Although there is no condition that is immediately life threatening, the way in which the parents are approached and how the condition is explained to them is likely to determine if the family will need long-term counseling or if the parents will accept the ultimate gender assignment of the child. This is a condition where experience and careful consideration are essential and a condition where I recommend immediate consultation with a pediatric endocrinologist before assigning sex.

NORMAL SEXUAL DIFFERENTIATION

Normally, gender identity is based upon genotype, which will determine gonadal sex, which leads to phenotypic sexual differentiation, which determines social sexual role. If this progression is not followed and an abnormal phenotype results, during consideration of gender assignment, attention is given to whether fertility can be retained and whether physical appearance is incompatible with chromosomal sex.

Genotype

Genotype or *chromosomal sex* is 46XY for a male and 46XX for a female. The *Lyon hypothesis* predicts that one of the X chromosomes in a female is inactivated so that only one dose of each gene on the X chromosome is active (although a few genes on the second X chromosome are retained in the active form). This inactivated X chromosome appears as a *Barr body* at the periphery of the nuclear envelope on a stained preparation of cells scraped from the buccal mucosa (the buccal smear). Patients will have one fewer Barr body than the number of X chromosomes so that those with more than

29

two X chromosomes will have more than one Barr body (e.g., a patient with 48XXXY will have two), and those with only one X chromosome (45X Turner syndrome) will have no Barr bodies. Unfortunately, few laboratories are capable of performing buccal smears in a reliable manner, and few physicians have enough experience either to perform the buccal scrape correctly or to interpret the buccal smear results appropriately. Thus, the buccal smear cannot be used as a definitive diagnostic technique; a karyotype determination is the only accurate approach.

The *H-Y antigen* is a gene product coded for by a gene of the paracentric region of the Y chromosome that purportedly directs the differentiation of the indifferent gonad into a testes. The translocation of the H-Y antigen to an autosome or the X chromosome can cause an XX individual to develop testicular tissue. Recently, a *testes determining factor (TDF)*, found on the Y chromosome but quite distinct from the H-Y antigen, has been suggested to be that true agent that dictates testicular differentiation.

Gonadal Sex

Gonadal sex is determined by the presence or absence of the H-Y antigen or TDF. The indifferent gonad passively becomes an ovary (in the absence of the H-Y antigen or TDF) or a testes in the presence of the H-Y antigen or TDF. If there is only one X chromosome and no H-Y antigen or TDF, the gonad will become an ovary during the fetal period only to degenerate into a "streak gonad" due to the atrophy of the ovum and follicles.

The steroid metabolism of the gonad uses many enzymes to convert cholesterol into androgens or estrogens; several of the enzymes are also important in the adrenal gland so that a genetic defect in an enzyme may affect both gonadal and adrenal function. Several enzymes are of the mitochondrial cytochrome P450 classification.

Phenotypic Sex

Phenotypic development is divided into internal duct development and external genital development. These two areas may develop in alternative directions.

Internal genital ducts are masculine if derived from the *wolffian ducts* or feminine if derived from the *müllerian ducts*. In the presence of the testicular peptide product, *müllerian duct inhibitory factor (MIF)*, the müllerian ducts will atrophy; in the absence of MIF the uterus, oviducts, and the upper two-thirds of the vagina will develop spontaneously. Dysgenetic testes may have more Leydig cell function and testosterone production than MIF production, and some level of muellerian development may occur. In the presence of high local concentrations of testosterone, the wolffian ducts will develop into epididymis, vas deferens, and seminal vesicles. As the testosterone and MIF will come from a testis, a unilateral testis in a true hermaphrodite could produce müllerian regression and wolffian differentiation on the ipsilateral side, whereas a contralateral ovary could allow the development of contralateral oviduct and a hemi-uterus.

External genitalia are bipotential until 8 to 9 weeks', gestation. Without intervention, the genital tubercle will become a clitoris, the urogenital folds will become the labia minora, and the labia majora will form from the labioscrotal swelling. In the presence of systemic circulating testosterone, which is locally converted into dihydro-testosterone (DHT) by the 5 α-reductase enzyme in the sexual skin, a boy will be virilized. The genital tubercle will become a clitoris unless DHT causes differentiation of a penis with fusion of the urogenital slit to cause a penile urethra and fusion of the labio-scrotal folds to produce a scrotum.

The fetal testes must be functional to allow the steps of virilization to progress. In the first trimester maternal human chorionic gonadotropin (hCG) stimulates the fetal testes to produce the necessary testosterone. During the last two trimesters, fetal pituitary gonadotropins are necessary to continue testicular activity and allow further normal growth of the penis; if the fetal pituitary gland cannot produce LH, the penis will be normally shaped but small, with a length likely to be less than 2.5 cm (microphallus) as compared with a normal length of 4 cm.

Any interruption of the normal progression towards masculine development in a 46XY fetus will result in some degree of ambiguous genitalia. Any exposure to androgens at a sensitive time in develop-ment will cause a female fetus to virilize to some degree and also cause ambiguous genitalia. If the female is exposed to the androgen after 8 weeks and prior to 13 weeks of gestation, the vaginal opening may fuse posteriorly to become slit-like, and the urogenital slit may enclose at least part of the urethra; androgen exposure after 13 weeks of gestation will only enlarge the length and thickness of the phallic structure without affecting the vaginal opening.

Social Gender

Social gender is determined mainly by the surroundings of the growing child, but because the physical appearance of the child influences those interacting with the child, gender role is affected by physical differentiation. Interactions with family and peers will teach the child how to act within the expected gender role. While a body of research suggests some effects of prenatal androgen exposure upon subsequent sexual orientation, the effects appear subtle and a girl exposed to prenatal androgens, if raised normally as a girl, will have a normal female gender identity. It is imperative that permanent gender is assigned early, in the neonatal period, and appropriately so that no changes need be made later. It is difficult to change gender successfully after 18 months of age (except for the case of 5 α-reductase deficiency), and changes in gender at even a very young age may cause the parents to carry lingering doubts about the gender of their child, doubts that may come out in actions rather than words.

DISORDERS OF SEXUAL DIFFERENTIATION

Diseases Causing Virilization of Genetic Females
(*Female Pseudohermaphrodite*)

Congenital Adrenal Hyperplasia

An abnormality in any of the enzymes involved in the production of cortisol will, in the absence of feedback inhibition, allow increased ACTH secretion. The adrenal gland, unable to make the end product which will suppress ACTH, will become hyperplastic. Depending upon the enzyme affected, the adrenal gland may make uncontrolled amounts of androgens to allow virilization of a female or, because the same enzyme is affected in the adrenal gland as in the testes, cause inadequate virilization in the male. A defect of an enzyme in the pathway toward the production of aldosterone will allow sodium loss and the retention of potassium (see Appendix 2, Table 2-1).

21-Hydroxylase Deficiency

21-hydroxylase deficiency is the most common type of congenital adrenal hyperplasia, is the most common cause of ambiguous genitalia, is the most common cause for virilization in a newborn female, and one type of 21-hydroxylase deficiency is the most common type of genetic disease in human beings. The 21-hydroxylase enzyme is a P450 class enzyme with the coding for this gene located on chromosome 6 in proximity to the HLA genes; progesterone is 21 hydrodxylated in the pathway toward aldosterone and 17-hydroxy-progesterone is hydroxylated in the pathway toward cortisol. All affected patients have elevated 17-hydroxyprogesterone and the suppression of this precursor can be followed to evaluate adequate therapy. About 50% of patients have clinical salt loss and hyper-kalemia. Within one family, if a proband has salt losing, other affected children will also be salt losers; further, the affected children within one family will share the same HLA types.

Females with 21-hydroxylase deficiency will be virilized in utero and may have any abnormality of development including clitoro-megally, posterior fusion of the labia majora into an "empty scrotal sack," and lack of formation of the vaginal vesicular septum, causing a urogenital sinus. Thus a female will appear to be at any stage on the continuum from ambiguous genitalia to "male with undescended testes." A male infant will not appear obviously abnormal and may not be diagnosed until a metabolic emergency occurs while a female with ambiguous genitalia will usually receive immediate attention.

There are rarely any metabolic problems during the first days after birth in patients with 21-hydroxylase deficiency. Hypoglycemia does not develop in the immediate neonatal period, and *salt wasting* does not manifest until after about 5 days of age. The initial signs of electrolyte disturbance will be vomiting. The real problem with this chronology is that many children will be sent home by 3 days of age, before any hint of electrolyte problems occurs. Boys who look normal may be mistakenly diagnosed as having pyloric stenosis and even undergo unnecessary surgery; one diagnostic difference is that patients with 21-hydroxylase deficiency have high potassium and those with pyloric stenosis have low potassium and metabolic alkalosis. If untreated, salt loss can lead to sodium values in the 110 mEq/liter range and elevated potassium to the range above 9.5 mEq/liter. Vomiting can lead to weight loss so that body weight falls to a point lower than birth weight. Simple virilized patients have no obvious salt loss but may have elevated *plasma renin activities (PRA)*, suggesting the need for extra salt or mineralo-corticoid therapy.

Skin pigmentation may increase during the period that the patient is untreated due to extremely elevated ACTH secretion. Androgen secretion will lead to *incomplete sexual precocity* in affected children with the appearance of pubic hair, clitoral or penile enlargement, acne, deepening of the voice, muscular develop-ment, rapid growth and bone age advancement. Although the child will be large for age, the rapid bone age advancement will lead to early epiphyseal fusion and short adult stature. Testes will not enlarge in affected boys since the androgen comes from the adrenal gland rather than the gonads; rarely, *adrenal rest* tissue in the testes will cause nodular enlargement of the testes in untreated boys. Remarkably, the advanced bone age and exposure to androgens will mature the hypothalamic-pituitary-gonadal axis so that when glucocorticoid treatment is administered, which lowers adrenal androgens, true precocious puberty may occur (with testicular enlargement in boys) and further compromise final height by bone age advancement; true precocious puberty following exposure to excess androgens can be treated with *GnRH analogues* like any other cause of true precocious puberty (see Chapter 3).

Late onset 21-hydroxylase deficiency is a recently described condition characterized by normal phenotype at birth (i.e., no clitoromegaly or posterior vaginal fusion in girls) but virilization occurring years afterward. The *17-hydroxyprogesterone* concentrations will be elevated in the basal state or after ACTH stimulation. Female patients may complain of increasing facial or body hair. The incidence varies in ethnic groups with an incidence in Ashkenazi Jews of 1 in 500, making this disorder the most common genetic disease in human beings. *Cryptic 21-hydroxylase deficiency* appears to be a variant of the late onset form; laboratory values are identical but for some reason the patient does not experience virilization.

The Diagnosis of 21-Hydroxylase Deficiency is made by an elevation of 17-hydroxyprogesterone, the precursor of the enzyme that is deficient, in the basal state or 60 minutes after 250 μg synthetic ACTH (usually 1-24 Cortrosyn but never intact natural ACTH) given intravenously. Serum concentrations of 17-hydroxyprogesterone are elevated in cord blood due to the activity of the fetal adrenal and contributions from the mother's steroid metabolism, but values fall to levels of 100-200 ng/dl within 24 hours after birth. A neonate with classic 21-hydroxylase deficiency will have concentration of 17-hydroxyprogesterone in the 1,000-10,000 ng/dl range or higher. Methods of screening for 21-hydroxylase deficiency in heelstick samples taken soon after birth are available and soon may be instituted in many states' newborn screening programs. Prenatal diagnosis is available by matching the HLA type of the fetus (taken from amniocentesis or chorionic villous biopsy) to an affected sibling of known HLA type, by restriction length polymorphism analysis of fetal tissue or by measuring amniotic fluid steroid metabolite values.

Older methods of diagnosis include analysis of a 24-hour urine collection for *17-ketosteroid* as a reflection of adrenal androgen secretion (primarily DHA). Difficulties occur if a full 24-hour collection is not obtained; we have seen patients mistakenly considered normal on the basis of a 3-hour collection that was fallaciously low. A 24-hour urinary *preganetriol* determination, a reflection of 17-hydroxyprogesterone secretion, suffers from the same reliance upon a full 24-hour urine collection. In present day practice it is advisable to obtain a serum sample for 17-hydroxyprogesterone and to request that the lab treat it as a medical emergency; some laboratories will comply with such a request and analyze the blood within a few days.

As salt loss is not usually manifested until after 5 days of age, vigilance must not be relaxed after several weeks of carefully watching the patient's electrolyte status! The rising potassium value of a heelstick sample obtained in such a patient should not be attributed to hemolysis and a careful venous sample should be obtained. Further, a timed urinary collection should indicate low potassium secretion and continued high sodium secretion in the face of rising serum potassium and falling serum sodium. A plasma renin activity should be obtained to confirm salt loss, but such a test result will not be available for several weeks and diagnosis cannot rest upon this test.

Radiologic evidence of 21-hydroxylase deficiency will include an advanced *bone age* if the child is untreated for a period of several months (a simple virilized child will likely survive this long but a salt loser will become profoundly ill before this age) and an enlarging pituitary contour (due to basophil hyperplasia) on lateral skull x-ray if the patient is untreated for years. If an ultrasound exam in a newborn with ambiguous genitalia reveals a uterus, the patient will most likely be a female pseudohermaphrodite and therefore most likely be a female with 21-hydroxylase deficiency. A vesicovaginogram with careful technique using a rubber dam to contain the dye will determine the anatomy of the internal vaginal structures and whether there is absence of the vesicovaginal septum causing a urogenital sinus.

DIFFERENTIAL DIAGNOSIS OF ADRENAL ENZYME DEFECTS

DEFICIENCY	NEWBORN PHENOTYPE	POSTNATAL VIRILIZATION	SALT LOSING
20,22 Desmolase	Infantile Female	-	+
3ß-Hydroxylase	Ambiguous in XY	+	+
	Female or Ambiguous in XX	+	+
17α-Hydroxylase	Infantile Female	-	-
11ß-Hydroxylase	Male in XY	+	-(HBP*)
	Ambiguous in XX	+	-(HBP)
21-Hydroxylase	Male in XY	+	+(50%)
	Ambiguous in XX	+	+(50%)

*HBP = Hypertension

   The Treatment of 21-Hydroxylase Deficiency Virilizing 21-hydroxylase deficiency is treated with *glucocorticoid replacement,* and the best approach is the use of natural compounds such as hydrocortisone (cortisol) or cortisone acetate (which must be metabolized into cortisol); synthetic glucocorticoids such as prednisone, prednisolone, or dexamethasone have their place in the treatment of older persons, but growing children are more likely to maintain a better growth rate with the less potent natural glucocorticoid. The dose is variable among individuals but for an initial dose, $18mg/m^2$ of cortisol or $25mg/m^2$ of cortisone acetate is useful. Oral glucocorticoids are usually administered in doses every eight hours, but in the neonate or a patient who cannot take oral medications well, intramuscular cortisone acetate is an alternative. Because the injection will last for three days, there is less risk of a missed dose with unreliable caregivers. A dose of 25 mg every three days intramuscularly is generally appropriate for a starting dose in a neonate, but the dose should be titrated to the child. It is important to remember that intramuscular cortisone acetate does not begin to exert an effect for several hours; it is not appropriate for a emergency, but only for long term therapy. If an emergency arises, subcutaneous, intravenous, or intramuscular hydrocortisone hemisuccinate is appropriate.

Many methods to follow up treatment have been proposed but the oldest, that of attention to growth rate and bone age, often is the final measure of adequacy of treatment; with too low a dose of glucocorticoid the growth rate is excessive because of excess androgens, whereas too much glucocorticoid quickly suppresses growth rate. Bone age advancement is determined yearly with an increase of one year of bone age for each year of chronological age the ideal. Serum 17-hydroxyprogesterone measured at a set time in the day after a dose of glucocorticoid (usually 2 hours after the AM dose in one scheme or at 8:00 AM in another regime) and testosterone concentrations are frequently used to monitor therapy; a 17-hydroxyprogesterone concentration value a bit above normal at 200 to 300 ng/dl and an age and sex appropriate testosterone concentration are the goals.

Mineralocorticoid therapy is administered to salt losing patients in the form of 9 α-flourohydrocortisone (*florinef*) at 0.05 to 0.15 mg per day orally (until recently deoxycorticosterone was available in the intramuscular and subcutaneous form but at the time of this writing, only oral florinef can be found for such therapy). Since the effects of mineralocorticoids at the proximal tubule level of the kidney are to retain sodium and excrete potassium, extra salt is administered at a dose of approximately 1 to 2 grams per day of sodium chloride; the parents may be given a few test tubes marked at the height 1 to 2 grams of table salt would reach so that they may measure the correct amount for the child. Blood pressure can rise high enough to cause hypertensive encephalopathy if too much salt or mineralocorticoid is given while too little will precipitate hyponatremia and hyperkalemia. Inadequate mineralocorticoid can also cause elevation of ACTH and therefore rising androgen concentrations. In such a situation where the body interprets salt loss as stress, misinterpretation of the androgen levels may suggest the need for additional glucocorticoid which would lead to growth suppression; if appropriate mineralocorticoid is given instead, the androgens will decrease and growth will normalize.

At times of stress, glucocorticoid therapy must be increased threefold. Usually this will be necessary when an infectious illness causes a fever over 37.5°C or 101°F. If the patient is vomiting and cannot retain oral medications, the patient should be evaluated at the office or emergency room but on the way, hydrocortisone-sodium succinate can be given subcutaneously, intramuscularly or, in case of emergencies causing shock and poor perfusion, intravenously. A dose of 25 to 50 mg of hydrocortisone-sodium succinate for a child under 5 years and a dose of 50 to 100 mg for an older child will be an appropriate initial dose for most emergencies. Too much glucocorticoid in an emergency is not going to cause a problem while inadequate dosage can certainly be ineffectual.

Patients with 21-hydroxylase deficiency require special preparation for surgery to avoid *addisonian crisis*. A dose of hydrocortisone-sodium succinate of 50 to 100 mg is given at the time of induction of anesthesia, and an infusion of the glucocorticoid is maintained during the procedure, or boluses are given every 4-6 hours to ensure a daily dose in excess of 45 mg/M^2, triple the secretory rate of the adrenal glands. High-dose glucocorticoid therapy is maintained during surgery and in case of complications, but in most cases the dose can be cut by degrees over the week postoperatively. Due to the risks of hyponatremia and hypoglycemia, normal saline is infused during the operation and as needed thereafter and dextrose is infused in 5 to 10% concentrations.

Patients with 21-hydroxylase deficiency can be treated in most ways like any other child, but because they can develop complication of minor illnesses quite easily, they must be watched closely. Frequent complications include hypoglycemia and hyponatremia in salt losers; any patient with 21-hydroxylase deficiency seen with acute illness must be considered to have these conditions until proven otherwise and initial fluid management must include dextrose and salt. We strongly suggest that patients with 21-hydroxylase deficiency wear an identification bracelet or necklace and that they or their parents carry an identifying letter from their doctor in case they require emergency treatment from an institution not familiar with their diagnosis.

Other Types of Congenital Adrenal Hyperplasia

11-hydroxylase deficiency leads to virilization, salt retention, hypokalemia, and hypertension; the enzymatic block leads to excessive deoxycortisol (compound S), deoxycorticosterone (DOC, a potent mineralocorticoid), and androgens. Glucocorticoid therapy is necessary to stop virilization and reduce salt retention and hypertension.

3-β-hydroxysteroid-dehydrogenase-deficiency causes salt loss and virilization in genetic females but inadequate virilization in genetic males. The enzyme deficiency causes an increase in dehydroepiandrosterone and its sulfate (DHA and DHAS) and elevated 24-hour urinary ketosteroids while serum 17-hydroxyprogesterone is low or normal. Treatment is as with 21-hydroxylase deficiency.

Other Conditions

Patients with both testicular and ovarian tissue are *true hermaphrodites*. The tissue is more often combined in ovotestes than distributed laterally with a normal ovary on one side and a normal testes on the other. Because of variable production of müllerian duct inhibitory factor and local and systemic testosterone, the internal ducts and external genitalia will be quite variable among individuals. Thus part of a uterus may be present on one side with some male ducts on the contralateral side.

Genetically the patients are most commonly 46XX, with the H-Y antigen or TDF present on some chromosome other than a Y. Other cases may be 46XX/46XY chimeras or 46XY individuals with a presumed 46XX cell line in the gonads.

Fertility has rarely been described in hermaphrodites, but the ovarian tissue can produce some feminization at puberty in some cases. On the other hand, the dysgenetic testicular tissue can undergo malignant degeneration and should be removed. Due to concerns over the difficulty of plastic reconstruction of the phallus, most patients are raised as girls.

Maternal ingestion of androgens such as progestins of androgen derivation (present oral contraceptives do not contain these substances) can cause virilization of female fetuses in some cases. Other cases of *dysmorphic syndromes* can cause ambiguous genitalia without noticeable elevated androgens.

Disorders Causing Inadequate Virilization of a Genetic Male
(Male Pseudohermaphroditism)

An inability to produce testosterone, an inability to convert testosterone to dihydrotestosterone in the sexual skin, or a resistance to androgen action all can cause male *pseudohermaphroditism*.

Testicular Enzyme Defects

Testicular enzyme deficiencies include some disorders in which the same enzymes are deficient in the testes as in the adrenal glands.

Cholesterol side chain cleavage enzyme deficiency or *20,22-desmolase deficiency* leads to the absence of all adrenal and gonadal steroid production and large, lipid-laden adrenal glands which may inferiorly displace the kidneys (the condition is also called *lipoid adrenal hyperplasia*). In the complete form, 46 XX and 46 XY individuals will have a normal female phenotype and no progression of secondary sexual development at puberty; in the incomplete form 46 XY patients will have some degree of ambiguous genitalia. Profound addisonian crisis will occur at 5-7 days after birth because of the complete absence of mineralocorticoids and glucocorticoids. Treatment is as for 21-hydroxylase deficiency with the exception that glucocorticoid replacement dosage may be less because of the lack of necessity to suppress androgenic substances produced by the adrenal glands of the 21-hydroxylase deficient patient.

17-α-hydroxylase deficiency eliminates the 17-hydroxylation of progesterone and pregnenolone and interferes with the production of cortisol and sex steroids; 46XX and 46XY patients cannot produce cortisol or androgens or estrogens but make excessive mineralocorticoid in the form of desoxycorticosterone. Phenotype is immature female in the complete form, but some incompletely affected males may have ambiguous genitalia. Thus hypertension, hypokalemia, and elevated serum progesterone, pregnenolone, corticosterone, and DOC but decreased PRA, 17-hydroxyprogesterone, and aldosterone in an immature female are the clinical cornerstones.

Other Enzyme Deficiencies Involving the Testes but not the Adrenal Gland

17-β-hydroxysteroid oxidoreductase deficiency interferes with the conversion of androstenedione to testosterone and estrone to estradiol. Phenotype is infantile female or some degree of ambiguous genitalia. Internal ducts are wolffian because of the presence of müllerian duct inhibitory factor. The upper portion of the vagina is absent (as a müllerian derivative) and the testes are internal or labial; patients have had "hernias" repaired that contained the testes without the correct diagnosis made. Gynecomastia or some virilization may occur at the time of puberty.

17,20-desmolase deficiency stops the conversion of 17-hydroxy-progesterone to androstenedione and 17-hydroxypregnenolone to dehydroepiandrosterone and thereby limits the production of testosterone. Phenotype is infantile female or ambiguous genitalia with undescended or labial testes. Some virilization may occur at puberty.

Other Defects Involving the Testes

XY gonadal dysgenesis combines a normal genotype with abnormal development of the testes so that both MIF and testosterone production are impaired. Phenotype may be female or ambiguous and internal ducts may be partially müllerian. Because of the dysgenetic testes, the possibility of neoplastic degeneration arises; gonadectomy is indicated.

Dysgenetic testicular development in XY or XO/XY gonadal dysgenesis causes low testosterone production and the absence of

MIF so that external genitalia are ambiguous and internal ducts may be müllerian with some wolffian elements.

Defects Not Involving the Testes

5 α-reductase deficiency reduces the conversion of testosterone to dihydrotestosterone in the sexual skin causing the formation of chordee (ventral binding of the phallus by attached skin), small phallic structure, hypospadias, bifid scrotum, usually with undescended testes, and a urogenital sinus. The production of MIF insures the absence of müllerian derivatives but the presence of testosterone itself supports the development of wolffian structures. At puberty, possibly due to rising production of testosterone, DHT dependent changes such as enlargement of the penis, descent of the testes, and pigmentation of the scrotum occur as well as increased muscle mass and deepening of the voice. There is, however, no appearance of acne or recession of hair. Most remarkably the patients are initially raised as girls in the Dominican Republic, where the syndrome was studied, but at the time of puberty and thereafter are considered male in social contexts. This phenomenon has been considered an example of the plasticity of human gender roles, but in all other conditions, the conventional wisdom is that a change in gender assignment, if necessary, is extremely difficult after 18 months of age.

The *complete syndrome of androgen resistance (testicular feminization)* does not actually present as ambiguous genitalia since in the absence of testosterone action the phenotype is infantile female. Internal ducts are hypoplastic wolffian ducts and the vaginal pouch is blind due to the absence of the upper 2/3 normally derived from müllerian elements. At puberty, the unopposed estradiol causes normal feminization, but the lack of androgen action eliminates the development of pubic and axillary hair. The defect is transmitted as an X-linked trait and is characterized by a decrease in the testosterone and dihydrotestosterone receptors or a postreceptor defect in them.

The *incomplete syndrome of androgen resistance* is due to a less severe deficiency or defect in the receptors for testosterone and dihydrotestosterone. Phenotype may be normal (with the only abnormality being infertility), may be underdeveloped male with small but normally formed phallus, or may be ambiguous. Internal ducts are male due to normal production of müllerian duct inhibitory factor. At puberty, some degree of gynecomastia may be noted and some pubic and axillary hair development should occur. Serum LH and testosterone concentrations are above normal.

Unresponsiveness to hCG and LH is associated with low testosterone production and ambiguous genitalia.

The Diagnosis and Treatment of Ambiguous Genitalia

Ambiguous genitalia in a neonate must be treated as an emergency. No suggestion of gender must be made to the parents until a diagnosis is established. It is appropriate to talk about "the baby" instead of "he" or "she," do not have the hospital print a card having any suggestion of gender on it and speak of "the gonads" rather than testes or ovaries. Never say that the baby is "partially girl and partially boy" as every child is either a girl or a boy. We tell the parents that the baby has a cosmetic problem, that the external genitalia are unfinished and that it is up to us, by the way of tests, to determine the sex of the baby. Even if the physician has a feeling about the outcome of the diagnosis, the risks of incorrect assignment of gender are great and it is best to support the obviously concerned parents without giving them false direction.

Steps in the diagnostic process will vary, depending upon whether the baby has palpable gonads that appear to be testes or whether no gonads are palpable (see Tables 2-2 and 2-3). While I will list appropriate steps, I must emphasize that in this case above all, the help of an expert consultant is necessary; even if the child's life is not in immediate danger, the vagaries of the interpretation of the tests could allow an incorrect diagnosis such as one in which a salt loser does not receive therapy or surveillance for hyponatremia.

The mother must be queried for a history of unexplained deaths in the family (which would suggest congenital adrenal hyperplasia) or for maternal androgen secretion or drug ingestion. The baby must be examined for phallic size (stretched length and width), chordee, the appearance of hypospadias, scrotalization of the labia, presence of palpable masses in the "labial" area, weight gain and growth rate. A careful rectal exam with the small finger to palpate for a uterus and adnexa has given way to the use of an ultrasound study for the same purpose. In an older child a bone age examination as a reflection of androgen effect is useful but in the infant will not help much.

Laboratory determinations will include karyotype determination performed as an emergency procedure (labs will hurry the process in most cases so that an answer can be obtained in 5-7 days) but no reliance should be put upon a buccal smear. Serum androgen metabolite determinations should be ordered including 17-OH progesterone, androstenedione, DHA, testosterone and DHT. Serum LH and FSH, if markedly elevated to the castrate range, may suggest dysgenetic gonads. Urinary collections for 17 ketosteroid and pregnanetriol are difficult due to the requirement of a 24 hour collection and although they may be attempted, the serum levels of androgens and precursors will be more important. These tests will take 5-10 days to return and the diagnosis should be relatively clear from the results. If a question remains whether there is a functioning testes remaining or what the activity of 5 α-reductase, an hCG stimulation test should be performed. The administration of human chorionic gonadotropin (hCG), 3000 units/m^2 intramuscularly should induce a rise in testosterone (or other androgen metabolites of interest) over 100 ng/dl within 72 hours in a cryptorchid patient; if the patient is in mid-childhood or older, one injection of hCG may not be adequate to stimulate the quiescent Leydig cells. If hCG is given three times per week for two weeks the testes may descend into the scrotum if the inguinal ring is not definitively too small: it is useful to measure serum testosterone (or other appropriate androgens or precursors) 24 hours after the last injection of hCG to see if testosterone secretion can be induced over a longer period of time. Serum levels of DHT as well as testosterone should be obtained if a reflection of the activity of 5 α-reductase is desired. If there is a question of testosterone responsiveness of the phallus, testosterone administration should be attempted (as noted in Chapter 3). Sexual skin biopsy for androgen receptors or 5 α-reductase activity can be sent to research laboratories for analysis.

The decision of *sex of rearing* in a patient with ambiguous genitalia of course depends upon the disorder that is diagnosed. One consideration is to retain fertility, if possible, and another is to ensure that the external genitalia can be made compatible with the sex of rearing. Plastic surgical urologic procedures, performed by an experienced surgeon, are required for any patient with ambiguous genitalia. In female pseudohermaphroditism the decision will be to raise the child as a girl in the conditions listed above. Most of these patients will have virilizing congenital adrenal hyperplasia and although their external genitalia will be virilized, they will have normal internal ducts and should have the opportunity for fertility if correctly treated with glucocorticoid and mineralocorticoids. The clitoris will be enlarged, usually too much to appear as a normal variation. The procedure of choice is clitoral recession with preservation of the glans and the nerve supply in contrast to the clitorectomies performed prior to the last decades. However, if the clitoris is too large or if the patient is non-compliant and it enlarges further, a clitoral recession may be inadequate to avoid pain that may occur with erection of the tissue and clitoral resection may be necessary. Clitoral recession is usually done by one year of age to avoid allowing the child to be noticeably different from peers in the eyes of babysitters or child care workers, since the child may not always be in the presence of the parents after the first few months of age. The vagina will have to be enlarged and the posterior fusion opened. If there is a urogenital sinus, the anatomy will have to be repaired as well. The vaginal procedures may have to be done in stages, with the final steps done at the time of puberty.

Male pseudohermaphrodites will usually have to be raised as infertile females with the exception of those with 5 α-reductase deficiency. Those with severe testicular enzyme defects or dysgenetic testes will usually have basically female phenotypes and can never make adequate testosterone while those with androgen resistance will never be able to respond to testosterone. Reconstruction of the phallus may be practically difficult or impossible. In all of these cases, the testes will be undescended or partially descended and will be subject to an increased risk of testicular neoplasm in a location where they cannot be regularly examined. Thus orchiectomy is the rule in all of these conditions. In testicular feminization, the testes will induce feminization at the time of puberty and may be left in until that time; the increased psychological difficulty of explaining the need for a gonadectomy to a teenage child will be encountered if orchiectomy is delayed. In 5 α-reductase deficiency there remains potential for fertility as a male and many patients have been raised as males after correction of the chordee and hypospadias. It is important to recall that if the penis of a boy with microphallus is responsive to testosterone, the child can usually be raised as a male; patients with congenital hypopituitarism may be able to achieve fertility with appropriate therapy.

Suggested Readings

Aynsley-Green A, Zachmann M, Illig R, et al: Congenital bilateral anorchia in childhood: A clinical endocrine and therapeutic evaluation of 21 cases. Clin Endocrinol 1976;5:381

Bardin CW, Wright W: Androgen receptor deficiency: testicular feminization, its variants and differential diagnosis.   Ann Clin Res 1980;12:236

Grumbach MM, Conte FA: Disorders of sexual differentiation. In Williams Textbook of Endocrinology. Wilson JD, Foster DW (editor). Philadelphia; WB Saunders, 1985, p 312

David M, Forest M: Prenatal treatment of congenital adrenal; hyperplasia resulting from 21-hydroxylase deficiency.   J Pediatr 1984;105:799

Miller WL, Levine LS: Molecular and clinical advances in congenital adrenal hyperplasia. J Pediatr 1987;111:1

Sternberg WH, Barclay DL, Kloepfer JW: Familial XY gonadal dysgenesis. N Engl J Med 1968;278:695

Styne DM: Sexual differentiation. In Handbook of Clinical Endocrinology. Fitzgerald PA (editor). Jones Medical Publications Greenbrae, CA: 1986 p 63

White PC, New MI, Dupont B: Congenital adrenal hyperplasia. N Engl J Med 1987;316:1519, 1580

Zachmann M, Prader A, Sobel EH, et al: A pubertal growth in patients with androgen insensitivity: indirect evidence of the importance of estrogen in pubertal growth of girls. J Pediatrs 1986;108:694

APPENDIX 2

TABLE 2-1

STEROID HORMONE BIOSYNTHETIC PATHWAY

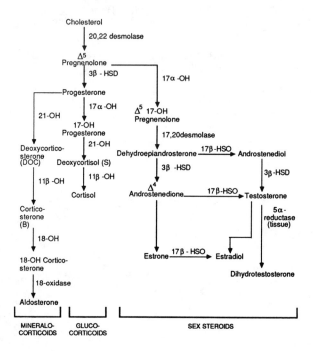

Reproduced, with permission, from Styne DM: Sexual differentiation. In: Handbook of Clinical Endocrinology. Fitzgerald PA (editor). Greenbrae, CA: Jones Medical Publications, CA: 1986, p 70.

TABLE 2-2

DIAGNOSTIC ALGORITHM FOR A PATIENT
WITH AMBIGUOUS GENITALIA
IN WHICH NO GONAD IS PALPABLE

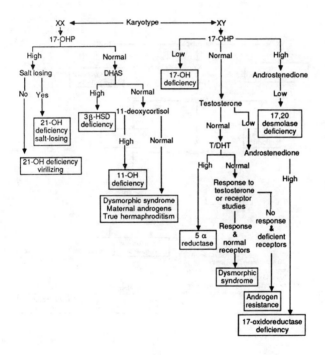

Reproduced, with permission, from Styne DM: Sexual differentiation. In: <u>Handbook of Clinical Endocrinology</u>. Fitzgerald PA (editor). Greenbrae, CA: Jones Medical Publications, 1986, p 68.

TABLE 2-3

DIAGNOSTIC ALGORITHM FOR A PATIENT
WITH AMBIGUOUS GENITALIA
IN WHICH GONADS (POSSIBLY INGUINAL) ARE PALPABLE

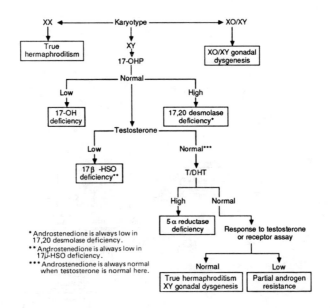

Reproduced, with permission, from Styne DM: Sexual differentiation. In: <u>Handbook of Clinical Endocrinology</u>. Fitzgerald PA (editor). Greenbrae, CA: Jones Medical Publications, 1986, p 69.

Chapter 3

Puberty

The striking physical appearance of secondary sexual development during puberty is caused by impressive changes in hypothalamic-pituitary-gonadal endocrine function. Puberty is best viewed as one stage in the continuum of reproductive function that actually begins during the fetal stage and extends through the climacteric. The age of onset of puberty is now stable in the developed world, although a secular trend of a decreasing age of onset of puberty has been documented until the last four decades.

PHYSICAL PUBERTAL DEVELOPMENT

The *Tanner method* of describing the stages of *pubertal development* is widely accepted. Objective description of physical development is essential to observe clinical progress.

Breast Development

B1   Prepubertal: elevation of the papilla only.
B2   Breast buds are noted or palpable with enlargement of the areola.
B3   Further enlargement of the breast and areola with no separation of their contours.
B4   Projection of areola and papilla to form a secondary mound over the rest of the breast.
B5   Mature breast with projection of papilla only.

Female Pubic Hair Development

PH1   Prepubertal: no pubic hair.
PH2   Sparse growth of long, straight or slightly
curly minimally pigmented hair, mainly on the
labia.
PH3   Considerably darker and coarser hair spreading over
the mons pubis.
PH4   Thick adult-type hair that does not yet spread to the
medial surface of the thighs.
PH5   Hair is adult in type and is distributed in the classic
inverse triangle.

Male Genital Development

G1   Preadolescent.
G2   The testes are more than 2.5 cm in the longest
diameter, and the scrotum is thinning and reddening.
G3   Growth of the penis occurs in width and length and
further growth of the testes is noted.
G4   Penis is further enlarged and testes are larger with a
darker scrotal skin color.
G5   Genitalia are adult in size and shape.

Male Pubic Hair Development

P1   Preadolescent: no pubic hair.
P2   Sparse growth of slightly pigmented, slightly curved
pubic hair mainly at the base of the penis.
P3   Thicker, curlier hair spread to the mons pubis.
P4   Adult-type hair that does not yet spread to the medial
thighs.
P5   Adult-type hair spread to the medial thighs.

Pubertal Growth Spurt

At no time following the neonatal period does a child grow as rapidly as during the *pubertal growth spurt*. Both growth hormone and sex steroids add to the increase in linear velocity during which girls gain an average of 25 cm and boys gain an average of 28 cm. The difference in adult height between men and women is partially due to the two year later age of onset of the pubertal growth spurt in boys compared with girls and due partially to the difference in height attained during the process.

Age of Onset of Puberty

The normal age of onset of puberty in North America is 8 to 13 years in girls and 9 to 14 years in boys. The time of transit from beginning to the end of puberty is also of importance because a delay may indicate hypogonadism. Girls complete puberty in 1.5 to 6 years with a mean of 4.2 years, whereas boys have a range of 2 to 4.5 years with a mean of 3.5 years.

Body Composition

Striking changes in body composition occur during puberty that lead to men attaining 1.5 times the lean body mass, skeletal mass, and muscle mass of women. Women attain twice as much body fat as men even though they start off with equal amounts in childhood.

ENDOCRINE CHANGES OF PUBERTY

The reawakening of gonadal function at puberty is known as *gonadarche*, and the increased adrenal androgen secretion is known as *adrenarche*.

Gonadarche

The pituitary gonadotropins, *luteinizing hormone (LH)* and *follicle-stimulating hormone (FSH)* are secreted in response to hypothalamic *gonadotropin-releasing hormone (GnRH)*. The GnRH is released episodically into the pituitary portal system in varying amplitudes and frequencies during different stages of development (and different stages of the menstrual cycle in females). If the pulsatile nature of GnRH secretion is altered to continuous secretion, the pituitary gonadotrope decreases its affinity for GnRH and the number of GnRH receptors decrease, which leads to a decrease of gonadotropin secretion (down regulation).

LH stimulates Leydig cell secretion of *testosterone (T)* in boys, and T exerts negative feedback inhibition of LH secretion; LH has little effect in girls until after ovulation occurs. FSH stimulates follicle formation and estrogen secretion in girls, and *estradiol (E2)* exerts negative feedback inhibition on FSH secretion. FSH has little effect in boys until *spermarche* (the onset of maturation of spermatozoa), when it supports the development of sperm.

In addition to their steroid products, both ovaries and testes produce a protein *(inhibin)* that exerts negative feedback inhibition on FSH secretion in both sexes. Inhibin is produced by the seminiferous tubules in males while the follicle of the ovary produces inhibin in females. After ovulation, the theca cells of the ovaries secrete *progesterone (P)*.

Hypothalamic GnRH and pituitary LH and FSH are present in the fetal hypothalamus and by midgestation, when the pituitary portal system is formed and hypothalamic peptides can reach the pituitary, GnRH stimulates extremely elevated secretion of LH and FSH, levels similar to those found in castrated individuals. In the male fetus, testosterone rises and is responsible for the enlargement of the penis before birth. Toward term, the gonadotropin concentrations fall.

After birth there is a period of instability when LH and FSH concentrations reach pubertal levels in boys until six months of age or more and in girls until 2 to 4 years. Elevated LH may stimulate T secretion in boys to concentrations greater than 150 ng/dl and peaks of FSH may cause girls to experience E2 concentrations in the easily measured pubertal range.

After infancy, gonadotropins and sex steroids are quite low until the *peripubertal period* (just before secondary sexual development begins). Children without gonads or sex steroids, such as those with Turner syndrome, have elevated gonadotropin values in the absence of sex steroids, indicating the functional nature of negative feedback even before puberty.

Quantitative changes in gonadotropin secretion are noted in the peripubertal period. Gonadotropin concentrations rise during sleep due to increased amplitude of pulsatile secretion every 60 to 90 minutes. As puberty progresses, the peaks of gonadotropins occur throughout the day until no diurnal variation remains in the adult. Gonadotropin values are higher in the adult than in the prepubertal child, but the pulsatile nature of gonadotropin secretion makes the interpretation of single values risky. If a nadir occurs during sampling, a different interpretation will be reached than if a peak is captured.

Sex-steroid secretion is more constant throughout the day than is gonadotropin secretion, but there is definite variation in estradiol levels so that concentrations may vary from 10 pg/ml to 40 to 50 pg/ml within one 24-hour period. Nonetheless, there is a stepwise increase in sex steroid concentration as puberty progresses. More than 97% of sex steroids are noncovalently bound to *sex hormone binding globulin (SHBG)* and presumably inactivated by this process. SHBG rises in girls during puberty due to estrogen stimulation, but values of SHBG in boys decrease. Thus, androgens in women are inactivated readily by SHBG, whereas androgens in men are relatively less bound and more active. This difference in SHBG, in addition to the higher testosterone values in men, accounts for the vastly greater androgenic activity of testosterone in men.

The rise in pituitary storage of readily releasable gonadotropin is reflected in the gonadotropin response to a bolus of exogenous GnRH. A 100 μg bolus of GnRH will cause a rise of LH greater than 16 mIU/ml in pubertal or adult subjects, whereas a far smaller rise is found in prepubertal subjects: thus, the rise in LH after GnRH is a useful reflection of pubertal status. Girls of all ages release more FSH than boys, so the FSH response to GnRH is not an adequate reflection of pubertal state.

Adrenarche

An increase in adrenal androgens is noted several years before the onset of rising gonadotropin secretion. The rise in the weak androgen *dehydroepiandrosterone (DHA)* and its sulfate *(DHAS)* occurs at 6 to 7 years in girls and 7 to 8 years in boys. The levels continue to rise through midpuberty. Control of adrenarche is separate from the mechanisms of gonadotropin stimulation; although ACTH must be present for adrenarche to occur, another as yet unknown factor must also be operative as well.

DELAYED PUBERTY

The term *delayed puberty* is applied to a boy who has not initiated secondary sexual development by 14 years of age or a girl who has not done so by 13 years of age. It is still possible for the patient to be among the 0.6% of the normal population who will enter puberty spontaneously at a later age, but by waiting until these limits to initiate a workup, the physician will limit the likelihood of performing an evaluation unnecessarily. Abnormalities of the hypothalamic-pituitary-gonadal axis may allow a normal age of onset of puberty followed by a cessation of progression; thus, patients who do not continue in their secondary sexual development also should be considered for evaluation.

Temporary Delayed Puberty

Constitutional Delay in Growth and Adolescence

Patients who are healthy but have a slower rate of development than average are said to have constitutional delay. These subjects will have a history of being shorter than their age-matched peers throughout childhood but their height will be appropriate for bone age. Their skeletal development usually will be delayed by more than 2.5 standard deviations. The body habitus will be thin. Although mental development will be appropriate for age, social development may lag behind if the patient has been treated as younger than actual age by family, teachers, and peers. There often is a family history of delay, so mothers should be asked their age of onset of menarche or other aspects of puberty and fathers their age of shaving (mothers have been shown to be more accurate in their memory of puberty than fathers). Secondary sexual development generally occurs when a bone age of 12 is reached for boys and 11 for girls. It is rare for a patient spontaneously to start puberty after the age of 18 years, and usually a permanent gonadotropin deficiency is present if that age is reached without pubertal development occurring; cases of spontaneous pubertal development are rarely reported after 20 years of age. Before that age, in the absence of a classical presentation of constitutional delay in puberty, it is difficult to differentiate temporary constitutional delay in puberty from permanent hypogonadotropic hypogonadism.

Various strategies of diagnosis have been proposed: a lack of rise in prolactin after thyrotropin releasing factor (TRF) or chlorpromazine is said to be more characteristic of hypogonadotropic hypogonadism than constitutional delay in puberty; a lower rise in LH after repeated stimulation with GnRH than after the first dose of GnRH is said to be characteristic of hypogonadotropic hypogonadism; and a rise in DHAS at the appropriate age of adrenarche in hypogonadotropic hypogonadism is described, whereas both adrenarche and gonadarche will be delayed in constitutional delay in puberty. Unfortunately, none of these schemes have proved completely reliable in individual cases.

Permanent Conditions of Sexual Infantilism

Hypothalamic Hypogonadism

Abnormalities of the hypothalamus or pituitary gland lead to lack of onset of pubertal development associated with low serum gonadotropins. If only gonadotropins are affected, the patient will be of normal height but may have *eunuchoid proportions* of long legs and arms and an upper-to-lower-segment ratio well below 0.9. If growth hormone is deficient as well, the patient's growth rate also will be decreased.

Isolated Gonadotropin Deficiency

In contrast to those patients with constitutional delay in puberty and those with growth hormone deficiency, patients with *isolated gonadotropin deficiency* are of normal height until the adolescent age range when, due to an absent pubertal growth spurt, they fall behind normal subjects in growth rate; because of delayed epiphyseal closure, they may continue to grow and reach a normal adult height. They have characteristic eunuchoid proportions with long arms and legs for the size of their trunk; this leads to a greater arm span than height and a lower than normal upper to lower segment ratio (0.9 or more is normal for adult caucasians). Patients with midline defects may have gonadotropin deficiency as well as other types of hypothalamic-pituitary disorders.

Kallmann syndrome consists of hyposmia or anosmia and gonadotropin deficiency. Within a family, there may be patients with disorders of smell with normal gonadal function and others with abnormal gonadal function and normal sense of smell.

Abnormalities of the Central Nervous System

CNS Tumors: Gonadotropins, as well as all other pituitary hormones, may be affected by *hypothalamic-pituitary tumors.* Late onset (as opposed to congenital onset) of pituitary deficiency, and particularly the combination of anterior and posterior pituitary defects, should suggest the diagnosis of a tumor of the central nervous system (CNS).

Craniopharyngiomas are tumors of Rathke's pouch in the pituitary stalk but spread to the suprasellar region as well as into the sella turcica. Tumors characteristically are found between 6 and 14 years of age. Usually, symptomatic, patients may complain of headache, visual loss, polyuria, and polydipsia. On physical exam, the patient may be found to be short, hypothyroid, and sexually infantile even if of pubertal age and found also to have papilledema and optic atrophy. X-ray, computerized tomography (CT) or magnetic resonance imaging (MRI) scan will show flecks of calcium within the tumor in more than 80% of cases. The tumor may be cystic and the sella may be eroded. Transsphenoidal microsurgery can be used for excision if the tumor is intrasellar. Larger tumors usually cannot be removed completely without causing neurologic sequela, but craniopharyngiomas are radiosensitive.

Other tumors of the CNS outside of the sella turcica such as *germinomas of the pineal, astrocytomas,* and *gliomas* (which may be associated with *neurofibromatosis*) also may cause hypopituitarism. Intrasellar *adenomas* are rare but may impair pituitary function.

Histiocytosis X (Hand-Schüller-Christian disease) may cause only diabetes insipidus but may also affect other hypothalamic hormones. *Granulomas of tuberculosis* or *sarcoid, postinfectious inflammation,* and *vascular lesions of the CNS* all can impair hypothalamic-pituitary function. *Trauma* due to accidents, child abuse, or, in fact, surgery all can affect hypothalamic-pituitary function. *Hydrocephalus* may cause hypothalamic-pituitary deficiencies.

Congenital Defects of the CNS should manifest in the neonatal period. *Optic dysplasia,* or the appearance of small pale optic disks usually surrounded by a dark margin, is associated with impaired vision and pendular nystagmus: this condition should not be confused by acquired optic atrophy, an ominous sign of a tumor. Approximately 50% of patients with optic dysplasia have absence of the septum pellucidum. Patients may be normal with respect to endocrine function, but any combination of anterior or posterior pituitary deficiencies can be manifest. Other midline defects, such as *cleft palate*, may be found in this continuum of endocrine defects.

Radiation Treatment, which includes the hypothalamic-pituitary area in the port, causes delayed onset of hypothalamic-pituitary defects. Patients with prophylactic radiation to the CNS during treatment of leukemia may demonstrate a fall-off in growth heralding the onset of growth hormone deficiency at an average of 18 months after the radiation.

Idiopathic Hypopituitarism

Congenital absence of any of the pituitary hormones may be found in *idiopathic hypopituitarism.* Because growth hormone deficiency itself may delay the onset of puberty in an untreated patient, it may be difficult to determine which patient has gonadotropin deficiency until the teenage years. *Familial hypopituitarism* may follow an X-linked or an autosomal recessive pattern.

Newborn males with growth hormone deficiency or gonadotropin deficiency may present with *microphallus* (penile length less than 2.5 cm). The absence of growth hormone or ACTH may lead to hypoglycemic seizures, and the combination of hypoglycemia and microphallus should cause immediate concern over congenital hypopituitarism. The microphallus can be treated with low-dose testosterone therapy (25 mg intramuscularly every month for three doses) to enlarge the penis without advancement of the bone age; sex reversal is generally not appropriate in congenital hypopituitarism.

Disorders and Syndromes

The *Prader-Willi syndrome* includes fetal and infantile hypotonia, short stature, obesity, and lack of satiety, almond-shaped eyes and characteristic facies, small hands and feet, deletion or translocation of chromosome 15 in some patients, mental retardation, and microphallus and undescended testes in males or delayed menarche in females. Some patients are described as being of tall stature during childhood with premature epiphyseal closure and short adult stature.

The *Laurence-Moon-Biedl* syndrome of polydactyly, obesity, short stature, mental retardation, and retinitis pigmentosum can be associated with hypogonadotropic hypogonadism or hypergonadotropic hypogonadism.

Weight loss due to chronic disease, malnutrition, and even dieting to less than 80% of ideal weight can cause hypogonadotropic hypogonadism.

Anorexia nervosa is a psychiatric disorder of disturbed body image associated with avoidance of food, regurgitation of food ingested, and performance of rituals around food (some affected patients may do all of the shopping for the family). Primary or secondary amenorrhea is frequently found in affected girls, and the onset of puberty may be delayed in affected patients. Weight loss causes a reversion of gonadotropin secretion patterns to the prepubertal, low amplitude pulsatile secretion.

Increased *physical activity* in the presence of weight loss, such as in ballerinas, or in the maintenance of normal body weight, such as in swimmers or ice skaters, may cause the cessation of menses.

Hypothyroidism will inhibit the onset of puberty and menses and, if hypothyroidism occurs after the onset of puberty, will stop the progression of puberty. Remarkably, severe hypothyroidism has been associated with precocious puberty.

Hypergonadotropic Hypogonadism

Hypergonadotropic hypogonadism is synonymous with *primary gonadal failure.*

Ovarian Failure

Turner Syndrome *of gonadal dysgenesis* is the most common form of *primary gonadal failure* in a female phenotype; the incidence is between 1:2000 to 1:5000 live phenotypic female births. It has been estimated that the 45X karyotype occurs in one out of fifteen spontaneous abortions and that 99.9% of 45X fetuses do not survive longer than 28 weeks of gestation. Classic cases have a 45X karyotype, negative *Barr bodies* on a *buccal smear* (this test has been replaced by karyotype determination in most laboratories), short stature, streak gonads, sexual infantilism, and a female phenotype. Other findings include fish-mouth appearance, ptosis, low-set ears, broad shield-like chest, wide-spaced and hypoplastic nipples, short webbed neck with low hairline, short fourth meta-carpals, wide carrying angle of the arms, abnormalities of the shape of the kidneys, multiple nevi, spoon-shaped (hyperconvex) hypoplastic nails, and left-sided heart anomalies (such as coarctation of the aorta). At birth, many patients have lymphedema of the extremities and loose skin folds around the neck. Patients have normal intelligence but may perform poorly on tests of spatial perception. Frequent episodes of otitis media in childhood may lead to conductive hearing loss.

Variants of Turner syndrome with positive buccal smears include mosaicism, such as XO/XX. Such patients may have some gonadal function and a more normal female phenotype. Sex chromatin-negative variants of Turner syndrome include patients with mosaicism such as XO/XY; since these patients may have dysgenetic testes rather than streak gonads and are at risk for malignant degeneration of the gonad, orchiectomy is indicated. Phenotype may be infantile female to ambiguous genitalia or phenotypic male.

Noonan Syndrome, or *Pseudo-Turner syndrome*, is a dominantly inherited condition with features similar to Turner syndrome (such as webbed neck, ptosis, short stature, wide carrying angle, and lymphedema) as well as features different from Turner syndrome (such as normal karyotype, triangle-shaped face, pectus excavatum, right-sided heart disease, and commonly mental retardation). Affected males may have undescended, often impaired, testes.

XX and XY Gonadal Dysgenesis may be sporadic or familial. Stature is normal and phenotype is sexually infantile female in the XX form or may be ambiguous in the XY form. Patients with an XY karyotype should undergo gonadectomy because of potential neoplastic degeneration of the dysgenetic testes.

Testicular Failure

Klinefelter Syndrome, or *seminiferous tubular dysgenesis,* is the most common cause of testicular failure, with an incidence of 1 in 1000 males. Due to variable Leydig cell function, testosterone levels in the adult patient vary from low to close to normal. Therefore, the onset of puberty is often normal, but secondary sexual changes do not progress. Seminiferous tubular function is invariably affected, and impaired spermatogenesis is the rule. In puberty or in the adult, testes are hard and no longer than 3.5 cm, with histological changes of hyalinization and fibrosis of the seminiferous tubules. Gynecomastia is common, a significantly decreased upper to lower segment ratio is apparent, and LH and especially FSH are elevated to castrate levels. Even before the onset of puberty, testes are small, upper to lower segment ratio is decreased for age, but arm span is equal to height, and many patients come to diagnosis due to personality disorders and mental retardation.

Variants of Klinefelter syndrome are reported with mosaicism of XX/XXY, XXYY, XXXY and XXXXY karyotypes. Other patients are reported with similar features to those of Klinefelter syndrome but with an XX karyotype (XX males).

Cryptorchidism *(undescended testes)* or *anorchia* *(absence of testes)* may be diagnosed in a phenotypic male with one or no palpable testes. There is an incidence of over 4% undescended testes in year one but about 1% thereafter, so descent of the testes may occur spontaneously in the first year; cryptorchid testes may have abnormal histology and even the descended testes in a unilateral cryptorchid child may be abnormal. The administration of human chorionic gonadotropin (hCG), 3000 units/m^2 intramuscularly should induce a rise in testosterone over 100 ng/dl within 72 hours in a cryptorchid patient; if the patient is in midchildhood or older, one injection of hCG may be inadequate to stimulate the Leydig cells and a longer course of six injections of hCG may be required, with testosterone determined 24 hours after the last dose. Further, if hCG is given three times per week for two weeks, the testes may descend into the scrotum if the inguinal ring is not definitively too small making orchiopexy unnecessary. GnRH has been used to promote testicular descent in European studies. It has been suggested that hCG and GnRH work only in cases of yo-yo or retractable testes which travel up and down in the canal and in which surgery would not be indicated anyway; in our experience hCG brings down testes in some cases where there was no indication of retraction before the drug was administered.

Orchiopexy is indicated if no descent of the testes occurs with hCG; it is felt that further testicular damage will occur if the testes are left in their warmer, intra-abdominal location. If no rise in testosterone can be induced with one to six injections of hCG, the patient probably has no Leydig cells and therefore has anorchia. The testes were present during fetal life to allow normal male phenotype and normal wolffian duct structures to develop, but atrophied, possibly due to vascular insufficiency occurring subsequent to genital development.

The Differential Diagnosis of Delayed Puberty

The first step in laboratory diagnosis of delayed puberty is aimed at determining if the patient has primary gonadal disease and hypergonadotropic hypogonadism or hypothalamic-pituitary disease and hypogonadotropic hypogonadism. If the gonadotropins are high, consideration should be given toward diagnosing a karyotypic abnormality such as Turner syndrome or Klinefelter syndrome or their variants (see Appendix 3, Table 3-1).

The most difficult part of diagnosis involves differentiation between temporary delayed puberty and permanent hypogonadotropic hypogonadism. If midline abnormalities are present or anosmia is present, the diagnosis is likely to be permanent impairment. If there is a compelling family history of delayed but ultimately spontaneous puberty (e.g., the father shaved later than his peers or mother's menarche was delayed), the diagnosis is likely to be constitutional delay in puberty. The presence of nighttime peaks of gonadotropins or a pubertal response of LH after GnRH suggest that secondary sexual development will occur within six months. Failing these situations, the patient must be watched for signs of spontaneous pubertal development or a rise in sex steroid concentrations.

Other strategies to differentiate temporary from permanent conditions have been attempted: the prolactin rise after TRF or chlorpromazine is said to be lower in hypogonadotropic hypogonadism; the response of LH to GnRH is said to be lower after repeated priming doses of GnRH in hypogonadotropic hypogonadism in puberty than in constitutional delay; a rise has been reported in adrenal androgens at the usual age in hypogonadotropic hypogonadism, but there is a delay in the rise in adrenal androgens in constitutional delay in puberty. Unfortunately, these tests have proved to be less reliable in individual patients than in large populations of study patients. Thus, watchful waiting remains the main method of diagnosing delayed puberty: if a patient has not gone through the changes of puberty spontaneously by the age of 18 to 19 years, it is unlikely that he or she will do so.

It must be kept in mind that if hypogonadotropic hypogonadism is suspected, with or without other endocrine anomalies, the underlying diagnosis must be investigated. Complete neurologic evaluation should be performed to uncover any indication of a CNS tumor. CT or magnetic resonance imaging must be considered if a tumor is suspected.

Treatment of Delayed Puberty

Psychological support should be offered no matter what diagnosis is established. The patient's immature appearance will cause stress and can lead to depression and suicidal ideation.

Sex steroids must be given to cause pubertal development in hypogonadotropic hypogonadism and may be useful in constitutional delay. In the frequent situation when the difference between the two cannot be established, temporary low-dose sex steroid therapy can be used in patients feeling the pressure of appearing immature who are not comforted by the thought of "waiting for nature to take its course." The goal is to cause some progression of secondary sexual development without advancing bone age and decreasing final height. After the age of 14 years (the upper age of onset of normal pubertal development), boys may be given 100 mg of *testosterone enanthate* intramuscularly every month for three months. If no sign of spontaneous puberty occurs in the three months following the treatment, another course of testosterone can be offered after the interval. Patients with known hypogonadotropic hypogonadism will have to receive testosterone therapy continuously in increasing doses until the final dose of 250 to 300 mg/month is reached over 6 to 12 months. Some men will require *hCG injections* in addition to testosterone to further pubic hair development and to achieve a more normal adult appearance.

Patients with growth hormone deficiency who have been treated regularly since an early age usually can receive this sex steroid treatment regimen. If they remain quite short or have not been treated before the teenage years, testosterone therapy may be withheld for a while and continued at lower dosage to ensure that maximal growth is reached before epiphyseal fusion eliminates the ability to respond to growth hormone.

Girls with delayed puberty may be treated with low dose estrogen therapy. *Ethinyl estradiol* may be made into capsules and administered at 5 µg/day for three months. If hypogonadotropic hypogonadism is proved, or if the patient has hypergonadotropic hypogonadism, 10 to 15 µg/day of ethinyl estradiol are given after feminizing effects are noted. After several months, estradiol is given only on the 1st to 21st days of the month. Usually withdrawal bleeding will occur each month after the end of the estradiol administration. After several more months, a progestational agent such as *medroxyprogesterone acetate* is given on the 12th to 21st day of the cycle. Because of the suspected increase in uterine carcinoma with exogenous estrogen treatment, it is recommended that a girl on estrogens have a pelvic exam yearly. As in boys, girls with growth hormone deficiency should not receive long-term or higher dose estrogen therapy until growth rate is normalized by growth hormone administration.

Patients with gonadal dysgenesis may benefit from new developments in the treatment of their growth deficiency. Previously, these girls were not given estrogens until the late teenage years for fear of decreasing their final height; presently, low-dose estrogens are started earlier to allow secondary sexual development at an appropriate age, such as 13 years, and to reduce psychosocial pressure.

Estrogen in low doses can stimulate growth while high doses of estrogen inhibit growth. Recent studies with *recombinant-DNA derived growth hormone (hGH)* indicate that growth rate can be increased in Turner syndrome with administration of double the standard dose of GH. The increased velocity is maintained for only one to two years, but addition of *oxandrolone*, a weak androgen, allows the effect to continue at least three years. The problems are the side effects of oxandrolone, including the growth of pubic hair, enlargement of the clitoris, and lowering of the voice. Studies are now under way to determine if low-dose estrogen is useful in addition to hGH therapy in Turner syndrome. At present these protocols are experimental and not in general use. However, it is useful to perform an hGH stimulation test in patients with Turner syndrome who are growing particularly slowly. Growth hormone deficiency can coexist with Turner syndrome but estrogen deficiency and obesity may combine to lower the GH response in patients to falsely suggest a picture of growth hormone deficiency.

SEXUAL PRECOCITY

If a boy develops secondary sexual characteristics before the age of nine years or a girl does so before eight years of age, the child has *sexual precocity*. If the etiology is premature maturation of the hypothalamic-pituitary axis, the condition is *true* or *central precocious puberty*; if the etiology is autonomous secretion of sex steroids or, in boys, autonomous secretion of hCG, the condition is *incomplete precocious puberty*. Patients will experience rapid growth and skeletal maturation and without treatment may fulfill the paradox of the tall child who ceases growing early and becomes a short adult.

True or Complete Precocious Puberty

Constitutional Precocious Puberty

Because of the gaussian curve that describes the onset of pubertal development, some children normally begin puberty before the lower age limits of eight years for girls and nine years for boys, without evidence of a disorder. There may be a family tendency toward this situation.

Idiopathic Precocious Puberty

If no tumor or other definitive diagnosis is found, the diagnosis of exclusion is idiopathic precocious puberty. These patients manifest all of the endocrine findings of normal puberty. Their progress may be rapid and continuous or slow and waxing and waning. Boys with this condition will first demonstrate testicular enlargement. Girls are brought for evaluation of idiopathic precocious puberty more often than boys.

Central Nervous System Disorders

CNS tumors are found more often in boys with precocious puberty than in girls. *Hamartomas of the tuber cinereum* are being found more frequently in patients due to the new noninvasive and sensitive CT and MRI procedures available. Prior to such techniques some of these patients would have had the diagnosis of "idiopathic precocious puberty." Hamartomas are not progressive tumors, and due to their sensitive location, are not amenable to surgical removal: medical therapy with GnRH agonists is the treatment of choice. Other more ominous tumors include *astrocytomas, ependymomas*, and *gliomas* of the optic nerve or hypothalamus. *Germinomas* may secrete hCG and cause incomplete precocious puberty in boys or may activate the whole hypothalamic-pituitary axis and cause true precocious puberty. Germinomas are radiation sensitive.

Other CNS causes of true precocious puberty include most space occupying lesions or causes of increased intracranial pressure, including *granulomas, suprasellar cysts, hydrocephalus*, or *head trauma*.

The McCune Albright syndrome involves the triad of cafe au lait spots, fibrous dysplasia of the long bones (cysts are notable on x-ray), and either true or incomplete precocious puberty. Other syndromes exhibiting increased endocrine activity such as Cushing syndrome and gigantism are found in McCune Albright syndrome.

Severe *hypothyroidism* can cause precocious puberty or, paradoxically, delayed puberty.

Any *virilizing condition*, when resolved, can trigger true precocious puberty, presumably due to maturing of the hypothalamic-pituitary axis. This may occur after instituting treatment for long untreated congenital adrenal hyperplasia, after the removal of adrenal androgen-secreting tumors and after the cessation of androgen therapy for various disorders, such as anemia.

Incomplete Precocious Puberty

Girls

Females can develop *incomplete precocious puberty* due to ovarian or adrenal secretion of, or ingestion of, estrogen. Gonadotropins should be low with slightly or significantly elevated serum estrogen.

Follicular cysts can secrete enough estrogen to cause breast development, and when the cyst resolves, withdrawal bleeding can occur. Usually cysts are small and limited in effect, but some can secrete levels of estrogen as high as tumors.

Estrogen-secreting tumors include *granulosa cell tumors* (the most common), *gonadoblastomas* (can arise in streak gonads of gonadal dysgenesis), *lipoid tumors*, and *ovarian carcinomas*.

Exogenous estrogen exposure may occur by diet (chicken necks and beef or veal may contain estrogen), or by ingestion of medications that may include estrogen (perhaps given to mother or grandmother), or even by contact with estrogen containing cosmetics.

Boys

Males can develop incomplete precocious puberty by autonomous secretion of sex steroids or by production of hCG, which will cause Leydig cell testosterone secretion.

Androgen secretion can occur because of *adrenal enzyme defects* involving 21-hydroxylase or 11-hydroxylase, *adrenal carcinomas*, *interstitial cell tumors of the testes*, and *premature Leydig and germinal cell maturation*. With *adrenal hyperplasia*, the testes will be prepubertal in size unless an adrenal rest of ectopic ACTH responsive tissue located in the testes enlarges in response to ACTH secretion. If the testes are the primary source of the testosterone, they will be slightly enlarged (over 2.5 cm) but will not be as large as found in true precocious puberty, but will not be as large as found in true precocious puberty, because the seminiferous tubules will not be enlarged due to the lack of increase in FSH secretion. A *Leydig cell tumor* will present with irregular enlargement of one or both testes. The GnRH test will be suppressed due to autonomous testosterone secretion in incomplete precocious puberty.

Gonadotropin-secreting tumors include *hepatomas, hepatoblastomas, teratomas* or *chorioepitheliomas of the gonads, mediastinum, retroperitoneum,* or *pineal gland* as well as *germinomas* of the pineal gland.

Variations of Early Pubertal Development

Premature Thelarche

Premature thelarche is a benign condition of unilateral or bilateral breast development, usually in a girl younger than three years of age. There are minimal or no other signs of estrogen effect (i.e., no dulling of the vaginal mucosa and little nipple development). Serum estradiol values are often low, as the follicular cyst thought to cause this condition spontaneously is often resorbed by the time the patient comes to evaluation.

Premature Adrenarche

Premature adrenarche is a benign self-limited appearance of a small degree of pubic hair, comedones, axillary hair or odor, usually after the age of six years. The normal rise in adrenal androgens such as dehydroepiandrosterone sulfate (DHAS) occurs earlier in this condition. Thus an eight year old with Tanner stage 2 to 3 pubic hair may have a DHAS value characteristic of a 12 to 13 year old. The rest of pubertal development, such as genital development in a boy or breast development in a girl, will occur at a normal age. There may be an increase in growth rate along with a slight advancement of bone age.

Gynecomastia

Gynecomastia is the appearance of breast development in a boy who is commonly in Tanner stage 2 to 3 puberty. In the majority of cases the condition disappears within one to three years, but in some cases it may last longer and require surgical removal. Obese subjects may have a reduction in the glandular tissue by reducing their weight. Pathologic gynecomastia will occur in Klinefelter syndrome, Reifenstein syndrome, or any form of partial androgen resistance, as well as in rare prepubertal boys with 11-hydroxylase deficiency.

Differential Diagnosis of Precocious Puberty

The patient should be examined to determine if there is evidence of true precocious puberty. A girl with breast development may have autonomous estradiol secretion or true precocious puberty; if a girl has breast development and appropriate pubic hair development, she probably has true precocious puberty because no other condition is likely to produce both feminization and virilization. A boy who shows signs of virilization with symmetrically enlarging testes is likely to have true precocious puberty although bilateral testicular tumors and gonadotropin independent Leydig and germ cell maturation are alternative etiologies; if the testes are not enlarging, another source of androgen is suspected such as an adrenal tumor or enzyme defect.

If significant isosexual pubertal development is noted (breast development in a girl or virilization in a boy), determination of sex steroid and gonadotropin concentration is performed. If sex steroids are elevated but gonadotropins are suppressed, there is likely to be autonomous sex steroid secretion. If LH is elevated in a boy, an hCG-secreting tumor is suggested as LH cross-reacts in the commonly used hCG assays and CT or MRI is necessary to look at a liver, CNS, or other location for the tumor. The GnRH test will reveal a pubertal pattern of LH secretion in central precocious puberty but will be prepubertal in precocious adrenarche or precocious thelarche (see Appendix 3, Table 3-2).

The diagnosis of true precocious puberty requires a search for a CNS tumor. CT or MRI is performed to determine if a hamartoma of the tuber cinereum or an expanding lesion is present; boys more often than girls will have a brain tumor as the cause of their true precocious puberty.

Treatment of True Precocious Puberty

Gonadotropin releasing hormone analogues (GnRH-A) are superactive and cause a down regulation of episodic gonadotropin release, such as is found during a constant GnRH infusion. Although considered experimental for the treatment of true precocious puberty at the time of this writing, they are approved for the therapy of prostate carcinoma. The effects are reversible and GnRH-A suppresses gonadotropin and sex steroid secretion, decreases the rate of bone age advancement and the rate of rapid growth, and improves the height prognosis of treated patients. Many university centers of pediatric endocrinology as well as the National Institutes of Health have treatment programs for affected children and can be contacted until these analogues are commercially approved for the treatment of true precocious puberty.

Medroxyprogesterone acetate (MPA) is a progestational agent that can suppress gonadotropins. It is not approved for such use, but in the past often has been invoked as a therapy for central precocious puberty. It is not as effective as GnRH-A in reversing the changes of true precocious puberty and has the side effect of causing a Cushing-like syndrome in higher doses and adrenal suppression even in low doses. It has been useful in the treatment in recurrent ovarian follicular cysts.

Testolactone is a blocker of testosterone biosynthesis and has been used in McCune-Albright syndrome in boys with incomplete precocious puberty and in gonadotropin independent Leydig cell and germ cell maturation. *Ketoconazole,* an antifungal agent, has a side

effect of causing a 17-20 lyase block in the testosterone biosynthetic pathway and also has been used in gonadotropin independent
Leydig cell maturation.

Psychological support is helpful to both child and parents. Their
larger size may make children with precocious puberty the center of
unwanted attention. Often children with true precocious puberty can
accept accelerated school placement so that they can be in a class
with children closer to their own size, even if their classmates are
older. Girls with premature menstrual periods should be prepared
before menarche and supported through this difficult time. Of
further significance is the possibility that the patient could be the
target of sexual abuse with the additional element of potential
fertility. Boys with precocious puberty and high testosterone values
will be prone to aggressive activity and may masturbate publicly, but
are unlikely to seek out heterosexual activity. In some cases the
treating physician can help the family through this stressful time,
but psychological counseling should be considered in the more
significant cases.

Suggested Readings

Cacciari E, Frejaville E, Cicognanai A, et al: How many cases of
true precocious puberty in girls are idiopathic?   J Pediatr 1983;
102:357

Marshall WA, Tanner JM: Variations in the pattern of pubertal
changes in boys. Arch Dis Child 1970; 45:13

Marshall WA, Tanner JM: Variation in the pattern of pubertal
changes in girls. Arch Dis Child 1969;44:291

Pescovitz OH, Comite F, Hench K, et al: The NIH experience with
precocious puberty: diagnostic subgroups and response to short-term
luteinizing hormone releasing hormone analog therapy. J Pediatr
1986;108:47

Rosenfeld RG, Northcraft GB, Hintz RL: A prospective constitutionally day of growth and development in male adolescents.
Pediatrics 1982;69:681

Rosenfield RL: Low testosterone effect on somatic growth.
Pediatrics 1977;853

Sklar CA, Kaplan SL, Grumbach MM: Evidence for dissociation
between adrenarche and gonadarche: Studies in patients with

idiopathic precocious puberty, gonadal dysgenesis, isolated gonadotropin deficiency and constitutionally delayed growth and adolescence. J Clin Endocrinol Metab 1980;51:548

Styne DM: Puberty.   In: Basic and Clinical Endocrinology Greenspan
F, Forcham P (editors). San Mateo, CA: Lange Medical Publications,
1986, p 456

Styne DM, et al: Treatment of true precocious puberty with a
potent luteinizing hormone-releasing factor agonist: Effects on
growth, sexual maturation, pelvic sonography, and the hypothalamic-
pituitary-gonadal axis. J Clin Endocrinol Metab 1985;61:142

Styne DM, Grumbach MM: Puberty in the male and female: Its
physiology and disorders. In: Reproductive Endocrinology, 2nd ed.
Yen SSC, Jaffe RB (editors) Philadelphia, WB Saunders, 1986; pp 313-
384

White B, Rogol AD, Brown KS, et al: The syndrome of anosmia with
hypogonadotropic hypogonadism: A genetic study of 18 new families
and a review. Am J Med Genet 1983;15:417

TABLE 3-1

THE DIFFERENTIAL DIAGNOSIS OF DELAYED PUBERTY

CONDITION	SERUM GONADOTROPINS	SERUM SEX STEROIDS	OTHER FACTORS
Constitutional delay in growth and adolescence	prepubertal (low)	prepubertal (low)	short stature but normal growth rate for the delayed bone age; adrenarche, gonadarche delayed
Hypogonadotropic hypogonadism	prepubertal (low)	prepubertal (low)	CNS tumor, midline defects or anosmia possible
Hypergonadotropic hypogonadism	elevated	prepubertal (low)	abnormal karyotype possible

TABLE 3-2

THE DIFFERENTIAL DIAGNOSIS OF PRECOCIOUS PUBERTY

CONDITION	SERUM GONADOTROPINS	SERUM SEX STEROIDS	OTHER FACTORS
Complete (true) precocious puberty	pubertal (pubertal GnRH test)	pubertal	normal testicular enlargement in boys
Incomplete precocious puberty			
Males			
Gonadotropin secreting tumors	high LH or hCG (positive pregnancy test)	pubertal or higher	moderate testicular enlargement
Leydig cell tumor	prepubertal (low) GnRH response suppressed	elevated testosterone	irregular testicular enlargement
Testotoxicosis	prepubertal (low) GnRH response suppressed	pubertal or higher	moderate testicular enlargement sex-limited dominant pattern
Females			
Granulosa cell tumor	prepubertal (low) GnRH response suppressed	elevated estradiol	sonographic, CT or MRI ovarian enlargement
Follicular cyst	prepubertal (low) GnRH prepubertal but FSH may rise above normal	low to high	sonographic evidence of cyst possible depending on time course

Chapter 4

Adrenal Gland

Disorders of the adrenal gland can lead to abnormal sexual differentiation, decreased or increased growth velocity, and life-threatening endocrine emergencies. Diseases can arise due to abnormalities within the gland itself, due to abnormalities in the control of the gland, or due to the ingestion of exogenous steroid compounds, even if for the treatment of bona fide diseases.

NORMAL ADRENAL GLAND PHYSIOLOGY

The adrenal gland sits above the kidney (which accounts for its archaic name, the suprarenal gland) and is composed of two major components derived from different embryonic tissues. The *adrenal cortex* is derived from mesenchyme and produces steroid compounds derived from the cholesterol molecule; the *adrenal medulla* is derived from neural crest tissue and produces catecholamines.

The median eminence of the hypothalamus secretes *corticotropin releasing factor (CRF)*, a 41 amino acid peptide that which stimulates the release of *adrenocorticotropic hormone (ACTH)* from the anterior pituitary gland. ACTH increases the activity of the enzymes of the adrenal cortex to facilitate the production of *cortisol* (*compound F* or *hydrocortisone*) which, through negative feedback inhibition, reduces the secretion of ACTH until an equilibrium is reached. Cortisol is a *glucocorticoid* that stimulates gluconeogenesis, helps the mineralocorticoids to maintain the circulation, and affects mood. Cortisol circulates in association with a protein, *cortisol-binding globulin (CBG)*.

The weak adrenal androgen, *dehydroepiandrosterone (DHA or DHEA)*, is dependent upon the presence of ACTH, but is produced in increased quantities by another factor which is poorly characterized;

this factor may be a pituitary hormone that is still unknown or may relate to a change in the metabolism of the developing adrenal cortex.

Aldosterone, the main *mineralocorticoid* of the adrenal cortex, can be secreted in response to abnormally high concentrations of ACTH but under normal conditions is regulated by the renin-angiotensin axis. Thus, in the face of lowered total body sodium or hypotension, renin, an enzyme produced in the juxtaglomerular apparatus of the kidney, acts upon angiotensinogen in blood to form angiotensin I; angiotensin I is transformed by the converting enzyme of blood and lung to form the octapeptide, angiotensin II; angiotensin II (and its metabolite angiotensin III) stimulate aldosterone production and secretion from the zona glomerulosa of the adrenal cortex. Aldosterone stimulates the reabsorption of sodium and chloride from the proximal convoluted tubule as, to a lesser extent, does its precursor, deoxycorticosterone (DOC), another potent mineralocorticoid.

Serum ACTH rises in the morning, about 6:00 AM, in persons on a normal daily schedule and cortisol rises thereafter. Concentrations of both ACTH and cortisol fall in the afternoon and evening as part of the normal *diurnal rhythm* of adrenal activity. If a person changes to another sleep-wake cycle, after a period of approximately seven days, the diurnal rhythm will normalize to the new schedule; thus, a person waking at night and sleeping during the day will have the peak of ACTH and cortisol phase shifted to rise just before awakening at night. Because ACTH concentrations vary considerably due to the *episodic nature of ACTH secretion*, a single serum ACTH determination may not be a valid reflection of the ACTH-cortisol axis. Cortisol concentrations are more stable than those of ACTH due to protein binding but can be quickly elevated by stress; unless serum samples for cortisol are obtained under relaxed conditions or unobtrusively obtained through an indwelling intravenous catheter, a high value may be specious. Serum cortisol concentrations, when abnormally elevated for time of day, are considered a reflection of stress.

DISORDERS OF THE ADRENAL CORTEX

Hypoadrenal States

The most common causes of decreased cortisol production are the *congenital adrenal hyperplasia* syndromes discussed in Chapter 2. In these conditions, ACTH is elevated in the face of reduced production of cortisol. Although the activity of the gland is certainly elevated, increased cortisol secretion is not realized and abnormalities of adrenal sex steroids or mineralocorticoids are noted.

Addison disease of glucocorticoid and mineralocorticoid deficiency is rare in pediatrics, but the findings may be mimicked by salt losing forms of congenital adrenal hyperplasia. Tuberculous infection of the adrenal gland was more common in previous generations and gave rise to most of the earlier reports of the syndrome. Autoimmune disease is responsible for the majority of cases of Addison disease at present, and often there are other associated autoimmune disorders such as diabetes mellitus, oophoritis, parathyroid or thyroid deficiency, pernicious anemia and malabsorption, hypogonadism, chronic active hepatitis, vitiligo, alopecia, or chronic monilial infection of the skin (mucocutaneous candidiasis).

Adrenoleukodystrophy (bronze *Schilder disease*) combines degeneration of nerves and the white matter of the brain and glucocorticoid deficiency with some cases also having mineralocorticoid deficiency. There is a defect in the metabolism of very long chain fatty acids and serum hexicosanoic acid (c 26) is elevated leading to an abnormally high ratio of c26/c22 fatty acids; experimental dietary therapy is being attempted as treatment for this progressively debilitating disease.

Congenital adrenal hypoplasia may cause an Addison-like condition occurring in an X-linked pattern, with a histologic pattern of cytomegaly, and may accompany hypogonadotropic hypogonadism. A recently described syndrome combines *adrenal hypoplasia, glycerol kinase deficiency, and muscular dystrophy* in an X-linked pattern. *Congenital unresponsiveness to ACTH* presents with glucocorticoid deficiency and may resemble the two conditions above. This syndrome has been called familial glucocorticoid deficiency and may be associated with autonomic dysfunction such as deficient tear formation and achalasia.

Adrenal hemorrhage in the newborn may lead to calcifications within the adrenal gland but rarely leads to compromise of adrenal function. Cysts and tumors of the adrenal cortex and medulla also may lead to calcifications within the adrenal gland. The *Waterhouse-Friderichsen syndrome* of adrenal hemorrhage associated with meningococcemia or other bacterial sepsis is rare but devastating.

Clinical characteristics of adrenal failure include increased pigmentation of the skin at flexural surfaces or areas exposed to the sun and at gum lines near the insertion of the teeth. Patients complain of fatigue due to glucocorticoid deficiency. Postural hypotension or an increase in pulse rate upon standing may be seen; a drop of blood pressure of 10mm Hg or an increase in pulse rate of 20 is considered significant. There may be a decrease in urine output due to the inability to excrete a water load. Salt craving may be noted upon questioning. Monilial lesions of the skin or nail will occur in the syndrome of mucocutaneous candidiasis and adrenal insufficiency, which combines an immune defect with an autoimmune disorder of the adrenal glands.

Laboratory evaluation of adrenal failure will demonstrate elevated ACTH concentrations at any time of the day and decreased cortisol concentrations when measured in the morning hours. Reduced cortisol reserve is noted on ACTH stimulation testing, metyrapone administration or insulin induced hypoglycemia (we do not recommend insulin induced hypoglycemia if the physician has no previous experience in performing it in children). Other signs of autoimmune phenomenon, such as Hashimoto's thyroiditis or diabetes mellitus, may be found.

Iatrogenic glucocorticoid deficiency is caused by the abrupt discontinuation of glucocorticoids. This may occur after therapy for a glucocorticoid responsive disease or after the removal of a tumor causing Cushing syndrome. The suppression of ACTH secretion is the etiology of the condition, and it may take months for ACTH to rise and more months for cortisol to follow suit. The tolerance of a patient to glucocorticoid withdrawal is difficult to define, but if a child has been treated with glucocorticoids for longer than seven days, it is prudent to wean the child off slowly rather than cutting the therapy acutely. The dose may be decreased rapidly until the physiologic range is reached; e.g., for a child on 20 to 30 mg of prednisone divided into two doses per day (which is equivalent in bioactivity to 120 to 160 mg of cortisol) for over two months, the dose may be cut to 15 mg for one week, to 10 mg for one week, to 5 mg for two weeks, and then switched to 20 mg of hydrocortisone (divided into two doses per day) for one week, 10 mg for one week, and then the medication may be discontinued altogether. A patient with Cushing syndrome or Cushing disease will be hypoadrenal when the glucocorticoid is discontinued via surgical removal of the tumor involved and a schedule of weaning must be followed; in the case of these tumors, however, the child may have experienced the hyperadrenal state for years, and the time of weaning from the high concentration of cortisol may be extended to several more months. Symptoms such as lethargy and headache and signs such as hypotension and hypoglycemia will indicate a weaning schedule that is too rapid. An ACTH stimulation test, a metyrapone test or (only if there is clinical experience in performing it) an insulin induced hypoglycemia test may be used to demonstrate ACTH reserve. Stress dosage of glucocorticoids must be given if the child has an illness or accident or if surgery is required (see Chapter 12).

Deficiency of ACTH or CRF can occur from a congenital defect; usually there is an associated deficiency of other anterior pituitary hormones. Hypothalamic-pituitary tumors can also cause impairment of CRF or ACTH function, generally with defects of other hormones (see Chapter 8.)

Hyperadrenal States

Cushing Syndrome

Cushing syndrome refers to the general class of hypercortisolemic disorders including those due to exogenous glucocorticoid intake. The specific causes include hypercortisolism secondary to increased pituitary ACTH secretion, ectopic ACTH secretion, and autonomous cortisol secretion by the adrenal gland. It has been stated that before the age of six or seven years the usual cause of Cushing syndrome is a adrenal tumor, and thereafter pituitary adenomas become more common. Recent studies suggest a higher incidence than suspected of pituitary etiologies for Cushing syndrome in younger children.

An abnormal regulation of the pituitary-adrenal axis leads to the specific diagnosis of *Cushing disease* (called *bilateral adrenal hyperplasia*, due to the enlarged appearance of the adrenal glands, even though the etiology is in the hypothalamic-pituitary axis). The original report by Cushing describes a patient with a basophilic adenoma and physical signs of hypercortisolism, but it was not until 50 years later that the primary importance of the pituitary micro-adenomas in these patients was proved by the technique of trans-sphenoidal microadenomectomy. The fact that some patients appropriately treated with microadenomectomy have recurrences suggests that hypothalamic CRF may be the etiologic agent for the formation of microadenomas, although a competing view is that the pituitary cells are primarily responsible.

Cushing disease in childhood first manifests itself with growth failure and is quickly followed by weight gain in the truncal or centripetal pattern with thin and weak extremities. Other features may include the classic Cushingoid appearance of a buffalo hump of adipose tissue on the back of the neck, purple striae of the trunk due to thinning of the skin and exposure of the capillaries, some-times, but not invariably, pigmentation of the flexural surfaces and gums, weakness and lack of energy, and the early appearance of acne or pubic hair. The personality of patients with Cushing disease may be bizarre and some describe the children as obsessive. The blood pressure may be elevated in the diastolic and systolic. Because of the small size of the lesion, neurologic symptoms or signs are not found in Cushing disease unless it has progressed markedly.

Autonomous cortisol secretion may be seen in single or multiple *autonomous nodules of the adrenal gland*(s) or in *adrenal carcinoma*. Nodular adrenal hyperplasia is characterized histologically by areas of active secreting adrenal tissue interspersed with areas of quiescent gland. A carcinoma of the adrenal gland often is difficult to differentiate from a benign tumor of the gland; pathologic criteria are available but often clinical observation is necessary to define the difference between a carcinoma and an adenoma. Carcinomas of the adrenal gland may have defects in 3 ß-hydroxylase and secrete large amounts of DHA as well as cortisol leading to a greater amount of virilization than in other causes of Cushing syndrome. Testosterone may be produced directly by such tumors, and severe virilization has been seen; the differential diagnosis should include virilizing ovarian tumors as well. *Feminizing tumors of the adrenal gland* have been rarely reported in childhood.

Ectopic secretion of ACTH is exceedingly rare in childhood but has been reported in Wilm tumors and in islet cell carcinoma of the pancreas. Serum ACTH may be measured above 1000 pg/ml, although modest elevations may be seen at first. The exceptional elevations can stimulate mineralocorticoid production leading to salt retention and potassium excretion; hypertension, hypokalemic alkalosis and subsequent muscle weakness will result. It is rare to see such excess mineralocorticoid production in Cushing disease.

Differential Diagnosis of Cushing Disease

Serum ACTH is not necessarily strikingly elevated in Cushing disease; the finding of a "morning" concentration of ACTH in the afternoon (ACTH concentration too high for the time of day) associated with a value of cortisol too high for the afternoon or evening is suggestive of abnormality in the regulation of the ACTH-cortisol axis. It must be remembered, however, that stress will elevate both ACTH and cortisol levels and can falsely suggest Cushing disease. As most patients with Cushing disease are obese, the differential diagnosis is often between exogenous obesity and Cushing disease. The *urinary 17-OHCs* and *urinary free cortisol* will be elevated in exogenous obesity due to the changes in gluco-corticoid metabolism of obesity but in Cushing disease the values will be higher than found in obesity (24 hour urinary 17-OHCs greater than 4.5 mg/m^2 and urinary free cortisol greater than 60 μg/m^2 are highly suggestive of hypercortisolism). The great variations in urinary values from day to day and the difficulty in collecting a full 24-hour sample of urine in childhood mandates that at least two baseline urine collections are evaluated and collected for glucocorticoid determinations. An *overnight dexamethasone suppression test* may screen patients for Cushing disease, but this test has not been adequately investigated for the pediatric population; one mg of dexamethasone is given orally at midnight and at 8:00 to 9:00 AM a serum sample is analyzed for ACTH and cortisol. In Cushing disease there is no suppression of cortisol or ACTH whereas in exogenous obesity the values fall remarkably.

The classic tests for the differential diagnosis of Cushing syndrome are the dexamethasone suppression tests. The *low dose dexamethasone suppression test* utilizes 1.25 $mg/m^2/24hr$ of dexamethasone divided into four doses per day for two days; if the urinary 17-OHCs on the second day of the test fall 50% from the two baseline collections (or if the 17-OHCs is less than $1mg/m^2$ and the urine free cortisol less than 25 $\mu g/m^2$), the patient is likely to have exogenous obesity. We find it useful to collect serum ACTH and cortisol concentrations during the baseline and dexamethasone suppression phases of the test to see if serum values also are affected (e.g., if the cortisol is suppressed to less than 5 $\mu g/dl$ and the ACTH to less than 25 pg/ml). If the suspicion of Cushing syndrome remains, a *high dose dexamethasone suppression test* is performed to differentiate between Cushing disease and Cushing syndrome of other cause. In the high-dose dexamethasone suppression test, 3.75mg/m²/24hrs of dexamethasone is divided into four doses a day for two days and urinary 17-OHCs excretion on the second day is compared to the two baseline collections; in Cushing disease there will be complete suppression of urinary 17-OHCs and free cortisol, whereas in the ectopic ACTH syndrome or with autonomous cortisol secretion there will be no suppression over baseline levels.

The use of *CRF infusions* for diagnosis is still experimental at the time of this writing. A patient with autonomous cortisol secretion will have low basal ACTH and will not have a rise in ACTH with CRF administration. A patient with ectopic ACTH secretion will have a high basal ACTH concentration and not have a rise in ACTH with CRF, whereas a patient with Cushing disease will have a large rise in ACTH demonstrating the responsive nature of the microadenoma.

Invasive sampling procedures more often are applied in adult patients than in children; if the technical expertise is available, however, these techniques may be applied to pediatrics. *Adrenal venous sampling* for cortisol or other metabolites may indicate whether there is a unilateral tumor responsible for the cortisol secretion or *petrous sinus sampling for ACTH* may indicate a pituitary or extra pituitary source for the ACTH.

Noninvasive radiologic procedures meet with mixed success. *CT scanning of the pituitary* region has not been helpful due to the small size of the microadenomas. The adrenal gland may or may not appear enlarged on *abdominal CT scans* in Cushing disease. A solitary nodule or tumor or nodular adrenal hyperplasia may be identified on high quality computerized scans or *magnetic resonance imaging* but this is far from certain and exploratory laparotomy may be required to localize the tumor.

Treatment of Cushing Syndrome

If Cushing disease is established, the treatment may be medical, radiotherapy, or surgery. Previous studies have demonstrated the utility of *o,p'-DDD*, an adrenolytic agent, but other methods have supplanted its use in all but inoperable patients. *Metyrapone*, an 11-hydroxylase inhibitor has been used with some success, but ACTH levels will rise and overwhelm the block in cortisol production leading to renewed symptoms of hypercortisolism. *Radiotherapy* has been used in some series, but the risk of hypopituitarism developing after radiotherapy has led most clinicians to use other methods of treatment. *Bilateral adrenalectomy* will cure the hypercortisolism but leave the pituitary tumor. After a period, the hypersecretory tumor, released from the suppressive effects of hypercortisolism, may grow and secrete increasing amounts of ACTH: hyperpigmentation and an enlarging pituitary tumor of *Nelson syndrome* results. This clinical course has led to decreased enthusiasm for bilateral adrenalectomy as treatment for Cushing disease. *Transsphenoidal microadenomectomy* is a useful method of curing the patient of the microadenoma that causes the problem and leaving the rest of the pituitary gland intact. Experience with this particular tumor is a must if the surgeon is going to remove the appropriate part of the gland. There is possible recurrence rate, but reoperation can be performed if necessary. In the right hands, this procedure appears the treatment of choice.

The aim of treatment of autonomous adrenal tumors and ectopic ACTH secreting tumors is to eradicate the offending neoplasm. If the ectopic secreting tumor is inoperable, an adrenal blocking agent or bilateral adrenalectomy is used to control the hypercortisolism.

The goal of medical treatment of Cushing syndrome after the correction of the hypercortisolism is the replacement of glucocorticoids as necessary without the suppression of growth. In the months after the removal of the microadenoma of Cushing disease, the remaining corticotropes will not function and replacement will be required. The initial dose of cortisol will have to be relatively high or the patient may experience the malaise and lethargy characteristic of glucocorticoid withdrawal. Although the desired dose of hydrocortisone is approximately 18 mg/m^2 and that of cortisone acetate is 23 mg/m^2, the initial dose may have to be twice that for several weeks, with gradual weaning to the lower dose necessary. Some patients experience headaches and feelings of malaise when weaned too quickly from the higher doses of glucocorticoids. After 9 to 18 months, normal adrenal function will return in the majority of cases of Cushing disease treated by transsphenoidal microadenomectomy. Of course, if the adrenal glands are removed, both glucocorticoids and mineralocorticoid will have to be replaced for the life of the patient.

Adrenal Medulla

Normal Physiology

The adrenal medulla produces *catecholamines* in its *chromaffin cells* and is derived from neuroectoderm. The other locations of chromaffin cells are the sympathetic ganglion and the organ of Zuckerkandl (anterior to the aorta) and although the extraadrenal chromaffin cells mostly disappear in the postnatal period, they remain a potential site of pheochromocytoma formation.

The catecholamine biosynthetic pathway proceeds from L-tyrosine to L-dopa (via tyrosine hydroxylase) to dopamine (via aromatic-l-amino acid decarboxylase) to *norepinephrine* (via dopamine beta hydroxylase) to *epinephrine* (via phenyl-ethanolamine-N-methyl transferase). The last step only occurs in specific sympathetic nervous tissue such as the adrenal medulla; the high concentration of cortisol in the blood supply to the adrenal medulla is thought to induce phenylethanolamine-N-methyl transferase and to account for the transformation of epinephrine from norepinephrine in this single location. The secretion of adrenal medullary catecholamines is dependent on central nervous system control. *Vanillymandelic acid (VMA)* and *Homovanillic acid (HVA)* are deaminated metabolites of catecholamines and are measured when excessive catecholamine production is suspected.

Disorders of the Adrenal Medulla

Pheochromocytoma

Pheochromocytomas are derived from the chromaffin cells of the adrenal medulla or the extra adrenal tissue noted above. They are rare in childhood but represent a curable cause of hypertension and must be considered in the differential diagnosis of high blood pressure. Further they are an integral component of the multiple endocrine neoplasia syndromes, neurofibromatosis and Von Hippel-

Landau disease and may develop after other components of the syndrome materialize.

Characteristic signs and symptoms of pheochromocytomas include hypertension (more often constant than episodic in children as compared with adults), weight loss, headache, vomiting, and, more rarely in childhood than in adults, paroxysmal episodes of tachycardia, flushing, sweating, palpitations or anxiety. Diagnosis is made by the demonstration of elevated urinary catecholamine, VMA, or total metanephrine excretion in a 24-hour collection. Plasma catecholamine concentrations can be obtained but may not add any information to the urinary collections, which serve as a reflection of the integrated catecholamine production over the previous day. Provocative pharmacologic tests are no longer employed because of the danger of precipitating a hypertensive crisis and because of the specificity of the plasma and urine collections.

Surgery to remove the tumor is the treatment of choice for pheochromocytoma, but the patient must be prepared for surgery and indeed for invasive radiologic studies by adrenergic blockade. Alpha adrenergic block should be administered before beta adrenergic blockade. Phenoxybenzamine is given orally (5 to 10 mg every 12 hours with increasing dosage until high blood pressure is controlled) for chronic therapy; intravenous or intramuscular phentolamine (1 mg per dose) is used for hypertensive crises which may occur while phenoxybenzamine is establishing its block. Beta blockade by propranolol (5 to 10 mg given three to four times per day orally) is added when the heart rate rises as the alpha adrenergic blockade is being established; propranolol may cause paradoxical hypertension if given before the alpha adrenergic block is established. If the therapy above is ineffective, alphamethyltyrosine (a tyrosine hydroxylase inhibitor) can be started at 5 to 10 mg/kg/day given four times per day. Surgical preparation also includes administration of salt to repair the plasma volume, which is invariably low.

An adrenal pheochromocytoma may be located by abdominal CT scanning or by scintiscanning with the synthetic catecholamine precursor, ^{131}I-meta-iodobenzylguanidine, which is concentrated by chromaffin tissue (at the time of this writing the agent is not widely available). If imaging techniques fail, selective venous catheterization and analysis of catecholamine efflux may narrow the search for the tumor.

Neuroblastoma

Neuroblastomas are malignant tumors derived from neural crest and are associated with excessive production of catecholamines; in spite of this, they rarely present with clinical symptoms of catecholamine excess (probably due to catecholamine catabolism within the tumor). They are often diagnosed from their size or the presence of metastases and have a remarkably high incidence of spontaneous regression. Urinary norepinephrine (not epinephrine), VMA, and particularly HVA and dopamine are excreted in increased amounts in neuroblastoma. *Ganglioneuroma* are benign, mature forms of neuroblastomas derived from sympathetic ganglion cells; usually silent with respect to endocrine function, they may manifest some of the signs of pheochromocytoma.

Suggested Readings

Bongiovanni AM: Disorders of the adrenal cortex. In: Clinical Pediatric and Adolescent Endocrinology. Kaplan SA (editor). Philadelphia: WB Saunders, 1982 p 171

Loridan L, Senior B: Cushing's syndrome in infancy. J Pediatr 1969;75:349

Phillipps AF, McMurtry RJ, Taubman J: Malignant pheochromocytoma in childhood. Am J Dis Child 1976;130:1252

Sisson JC, Frager MS, Valk TW, et al: Scintigraphic localization of pheochromocytomas. J Clin Endocrinol Metab 1977;6:779

Styne DM, et al: Treatment of Cushing's Disease in childhood and adolescence by transsphenoidal microadenomectomy. N Engl J Med 1984;310:889

Styne DM, et al: Endocrinologic, histologic and biochemical characterization of ACTH and calcitonin producing islet cell carcinoma of the pancreas in childhood. J Clin Endocrinol Metab 1983;57:723

Voorhess ML: Disorders of the adrenal medulla multiple endocrine adenomatosis syndromes. In: Clinical Pediatric and Adolescent Endocrinology. Kaplan SA (editor). Philadelphia: WB Saunders, 1982 p 199

Chapter 5

Vasopressin Metabolism

Excessive urination can be due to the desire for secondary gain, to habitual excessive drinking, to urinary tract defects in concentrating ability, to osmotic diuresis, or to a lack of antidiuretic hormone (ADH). The major etiology of pathological osmotic diuresis is the glucosuria of diabetes mellitus (sweet urine) while the lack of antidiuretic hormone leads to diabetes insipidus (weak urine).

NORMAL VASOPRESSIN PHYSIOLOGY

Arginine vasopressin is the human *antidiuretic hormone.* It is produced in the paraventricular and supraoptic nuclei of the hypothalamus along with the neurophysins to which vasopressin is bound. The magnacellular neurons terminate, for the most part, in the *posterior pituitary gland* (the *neurohypophysis*), but some terminate in the third ventricle and some high in the pituitary stalk or in the median eminence. An intracellular *osmotic detector* located close to the supraoptic nuclei but separate from the nuclei containing ADH detects changes in plasma osmolality of as little as 1 to 2%, reaching a sensitivity which is better than most laboratory osmolality detectors. An increase in osmolality due to dehydration, or the infusion of a hypertonic solution such as concentrated saline, triggers the release of sufficient vasopressin to retain fluid and decrease the serum osmolality to normal.

Stretch receptors in the right atrium and *baroreceptors* in the carotid sinus also regulate the release of vasopressin so that a decrease in blood volume of 10% (equivalent to a major hemorrhage) will stimulate a large release in vasopressin. Lung disease and respirator therapy will trigger vasopressin secretion due to effects on the volume receptor. In the daily routine of standing and walking, vasopressin concentrations change from moment to moment due to stimulation of the baroreceptor. Other stimuli to vasopressin secretion include nausea and certain drugs, such as chlorpromazine and antimetabolites, used in the treatment of cancer.

Vasopressin exerts two major biological effects: it increases permeability of the collecting duct to water filtered in the urine and, in large concentrations, ADH stimulates the contraction of arterial muscle, which raises blood pressure. The medulla of the kidney has a high osmotic concentration of urea and sodium built up by the countercurrent exchange system. When vasopressin allows water filtered in the urine to pass through the collecting ducts, the water will, through the osmotic gradient, be drawn to the medulla, and the urine will become concentrated. The effects of vasopressin on salt balance are mediated through its effect upon changes in water balance as vasopressin itself has no effect upon the transport of sodium or chloride. If vasopressin cannot be released from the posterior pituitary, *central diabetes insipidus* occurs. If the collecting duct cannot respond to the vasopressin, *nephrogenic diabetes insipidus* occurs. If a patient has been drinking large amounts of water for a prolonged period of time through *psychogenic polydipsia,* the medullary interstitial gradient becomes progressively more dilute ("washes out") so that maximal concentrating ability of the kidney is decreased and polyuria results. Infection or various types of kidney disease also can decrease the concentrating ability of the kidney.

The consequences of *hyperosmolality* or *hypoosmolality* can be severe. The obvious impairment of renal function due to severe volume constriction and the pulmonary edema and heart failure of volume excess are well appreciated. However, the effects of rapid fluid shifts on the brain are more devastating and permanent. A rapid rise in plasma osmolality can draw fluid from the brain and, especially in young infants, cause brain shrinkage and rupture of veins bridging the distance between the rigid cranium and the more malleable brain substance. Although the brain is slower to correct osmolar balance than the vascular compartment, during a more gradual rise in intravascular osmolality the brain can produce "idiogenic osmols" that increase intracellular osmolality to balance a intravascular hyperosmolality; these osmolar-active molecules remain in the brain for hours and days after a drop in intravascular osmolality occurs, leading to an imbalance of osmolar forces with the net shift of fluid toward the brain, resulting in cerebral edema. Thus, both hypoosmolality and hyperosmolality are damaging to the brain.

Diabetes Insipidus

Central Diabetes Insipidus

The inability to release adequate arginine vasopressin in the face of increased serum osmolality can be caused by a tumor, trauma, infection, or granuloma as well as by a congenital defect. Some vasopressin secretion may remain in spite of the disorder, but the amount of vasopressin secreted is not commensurate with the need for water conservation, and excessive urination occurs. Depending upon the nature of the defect, the sense of thirst may or may not remain intact.

Any *hypothalamic-pituitary tumor* can cause diabetes insipidus with or without other hypothalamic-pituitary disorders. Most commonly in the pediatric age group a *craniopharyngioma* or *germinoma* is involved. *Histiocytosis X* or *Hand-Schüller-Christian disease* is an infiltrative lesion also associated with diabetes insipidus. Thus, the late onset of posterior pituitary disease in the form of diabetes insipidus, associated with any anterior pituitary deficiency or not, is cause for a full effort to diagnose a tumor or infiltrative lesion. *Trauma*, whether accidental, such as a fall off a horse or an automobile accident, or iatrogenic, such as surgery for a craniopharyngioma, can lead to diabetes insipidus. Hydrocephalus also can lead to vasopressin deficiency and diabetes insipidus.

Idiopathic, congenital diabetes insipidus without anatomical abnormalities can occur sporadically or in a dominantly inherited familial pattern. Congenital *midline defects of the central nervous system* can lead to diabetes insipidus in addition to anterior pituitary deficiencies. *Optic hypoplasia* often is associated with hypothalamic abnormalities; initial clinical presentation may be a visual deficiency or an endocrine disorder, including diabetes insipidus. *Absence of the septum pellucidum* may be associated with optic hypoplasia and leads to the term, *septo-optic hypoplasia*. Histiocytosis X and cranio-pharyngiomas can occur in infants, although these conditions usually occur at a later age. Thus, the *early onset of anterior and posterior pituitary disorders* usually carries a more benign prognosis than late onset but evaluation for potential tumor should be carried out even in the youngest cases.

Nephrogenic Diabetes Insipidus

Originally *nephrogenic diabetes insipidus* was thought to be an x-linked disorder, but numerous cases of sporadic occurrence or autosomal dominant inheritance have since been described. There appears to be a defect in the adenyl cyclase system of the renal tubular cells, as circulating vasopressin can be measured in affected patients. Because the disorder is classically congenital, these babies are more prone to dehydration than the majority of cases of central diabetes insipidus. Severe dehydration may cause episodes of unexplained fevers, failure to thrive, and mental retardation; hypernatremia may be demonstrated during such dehydration. Usually, when the child reaches an age where water can be obtained ad lib, the symptoms will decrease except at time of illness, causing a decrease in oral intake.

Clinical Features of Diabetes Insipidus

Clinical features of diabetes insipidus of either the central or nephrogenic variety relate to drinking and urinating patterns. The patient will urinate large quantities throughout the day and night, awakening several times a night while constantly drinking cool water (usually, other fluids are not requested) due to continuous thirst. As noted, except for congenital defects, diabetes insipidus usually occurs after infancy. If infants are affected, they will cry if deprived of their bottle and may drink their bath water or suck on their washcloths; these symptoms may be more common in those with nephrogenic diabetes insipidus. Older children and adults will go to bed with gallons of water at their side for use throughout the night. These features are in distinction to the compulsive water drinker who usually will go through the night without awakening and the child drinking for secondary gain who drinks small amounts frequently and who urinates frequently but in small quantities. At times of disability or when water cannot be obtained, the patient with diabetes insipidus will become severely dehydrated and could go into shock. Due to the massive flow of urine, the renal pelvises and ureters may show dilation on intravenous pyelogram.

Diagnosis of Diabetes Insipidus

Before any assessment is made for diabetes insipidus, it should be established that the patient does not have chronic renal disease or urinary tract infection that can explain the symptoms. To suggest a diagnosis of diabetes insipidus, a urine sample should be free of sugar and be dilute. The first question of importance is whether the patient really is urinating frequently in large quantities through the day and night. The history should allude to such a pattern and observation in the hospital or under the observation of reliable parents should be the first step to confirming increased urine output and fluid intake. The first voided urine sample in the morning is normally the most concentrated of the whole day, and a sample should be subjected to analysis of specific gravity and osmolality (remember that specific gravity can be raised fallaciously by contamination with nonosmotic substances, for instance, stool). A serum osmolality and sodium should be obtained; in diabetes insipidus, the values will be normal or slightly elevated if the patient has free access to water and a normal thirst mechanism, while in psychogenic polydipsia, the values will be low to normal due to the dilutional effect of the water drinking. An ambulatory, conscious patient without a thirst mechanism will have a high osmolality and sodium because such patients do not have the normal drive to increase water intake with concentration of the blood volume; this condition has been called primary hypernatremia in some reports.

If the tests noted above still suggest that the patient has diabetes insipidus, a careful *water deprivation test* should be performed. The most important consideration of such a test is to observe the child constantly for signs of dehydration and for "cheating" and taking water surreptitiously; the test should be done only with full staffing, and no part of the thirst should occur at night when the hospital staff is reduced. The child must be expected to complain about lack of water whether there is diabetes insipidus or psychogenic polydipsia, and the parents likewise might be uncomfortable over the procedure as the child cries for water. The child should have a normal dinner, and the usual nighttime routine should continue.

The next morning, the first voided urine should be analyzed for osmolality, the weight and blood pressure should be determined, and a serum sodium and a hematocrit should be obtained. At that time a normal breakfast can be given with normal fluid and then all oral intake should cease. Weight and blood pressure should be taken hourly, serum osmolality and hematocrit every two hours, and all urine volume monitored and osmolality measured every void. The test should cease if the weight drops 5%, the blood pressure falls, or the osmolality rises above 300 mosm/liter. Otherwise, at the end of eight hours, the serum and urine osmolality should be compared and a serum vasopressin obtained to match with the osmolalities (the vasopressin value will not return for weeks from the laboratory but may prove useful if the diagnosis is still in doubt).

As a patient becomes dehydrated, the urine osmolality will rise due to the delivery of increasingly concentrated filtrate to the kidney, but a patient with diabetes insipidus cannot concentrate the urine to more than 1.5 to 2 times the serum osmolality. If the serum osmolality rises to 300 mosm/liter or higher, the urine should normally be more than 450 mosm/liter. In an intermediate situation where a trend toward dehydration is developing, a continuation of the thirst may be necessary. Further, in partial diabetes insipidus, a patient may pass just one test with adequate urinary concentration whereas, if the test is repeated the next day, the patient may be totally unable to concentrate the urine because of the exhaustion of the patient's meager supply of vasopressin.

If the serum osmolality has risen without concentration of the urine osmolality, a dose of aqueous vasopressin is administered at 0.3 ml/m^2 of 20 units/ml aqueous vasopressin subcutaneously or 0.05-0.15 ml of *d-arginine-d-amino-vasopressin(DDAVP)* in a nostril and in the next 30 to 60 minutes, the volume of urine and the concentration is compared to the values before the exogenous vasopressin or DDAVP. In central diabetes insipidus, at the end of the thirst, maximal vasopressin for the patient, but inadequate vasopressin for the task of concentrating the urine, will have been released so that exogenous vasopressin will significantly further concentrate the urine. If the patient has psychogenic polydipsia, because of excess water load the patient has taken in prior to the onset of the test, the serum osmolality may not rise much above normal during the thirst; because of the washed out medullary gradient, the patient may not reach full urinary concentration even if the fast is continued. However, the exogenous vasopressin will not cause further concentration of the urine because a patient with psychogenic polydipsia is perfectly able to release adequate endogenous vasopressin in the face of dehydration. A patient with nephrogenic diabetes insipidus will not be able to concentrate urine in spite of rising serum osmolality and the addition of exogenous vasopressin will not further raise urine osmolality or reduce urine volume.

Treatment of Diabetes Insipidus

A patient with diabetes insipidus, if given sufficient water, will be able to survive, albeit with dilated ureters and renal pelvises due to massive urinary flow. However, therapy to reduce urine flow is safe and available in the form of *DDAVP*, an altered vasopressin molecule that has 140 times the urine concentrating ability but almost none of the vasoactive effects of arginine vasopressin; a dose will usually last approximately 12 hours, whereas native vasopressin has a half-life of 20 minutes. DDAVP is administered in measured doses through inhalation by the nostrils, a method easier in older children than infants. A syringe may be used to squirt DDAVP into the nostrils of the youngest children. A dose of 0.05 to 0.15 ml is given and repeated when the child complains of increasing thirst or an infant begins to increase urinary frequency again. Ideally, DDAVP is given twice a day to make administration easier in school-aged children, but it is generally advisable to allow the patient to experience a phase of dilution before the next dose is given. A standing order of twice daily dosage is not optimal. In the presence of an intact thirst mechanism, the patient should maintain a normal sodium concentration. Patients with partial diabetes insipidus can be treated with chlorpromazine, which increases the secretion of residual vasopressin; due to numerous side effects of chlorpromazine, this therapy is not advisable since the availability of DDAVP.

Patients with *an absent thirst mechanism* and diabetes insipidus are extremely difficult to treat. A set regime is empirically determined under careful observation so that a given number of glasses of water per day sufficient to keep the serum sodium normal is prescribed. An extra glass of water should be given for moderately increased activity or exposure to high temperature. Every week or two the serum sodium should be checked, more often if stability of the value has not been reached. The consequences of dehydration or overhydration should not be minimized in this complex condition.

The treatment of nephrogenic diabetes insipidus seems paradoxical; a low-sodium diet and diuretic therapy is prescribed. With decreased serum solute due to the low sodium intake and the loss due to diuresis, the site of reabsorption of water shifts from the collecting duct where vasopressin exerts its effect to the proximal tubule where aldosterone, maximally stimulated due to whole body sodium loss, will attempt to retain all available sodium and thereby carry water back into the vascular compartment and decrease urine flow.

The Syndrome of Inappropriate Antidiuretic Hormone Secretion (SIADH)

In the presence of vasopressin and excessive water, the expansion of intravascular volume will cause a lowering of serum sodium and osmolality as well as a sodium diuresis and some degree of concentration of the urine; this constellation is physiologically paradoxical because the low serum sodium and osmolality could be corrected if the urine is maximally diluted and maximal urinary sodium reabsorption is accomplished. *Atrial naturetic peptide* may be responsible for the sodium diuresis as it is elevated in times of volume overload. Because the combination of vasopressin secretion and water intake is responsible for SIADH, the syndrome is often iatrogenic; the patient already may be under a physician's care and may kept on the same regime of fluid therapy after the vasopressin secretion begins. If fluid therapy in the treatment of conditions predisposing to SIADH is appropriately regulated and if serum sodium concentrations are monitored routinely, the incidence of SIADH would decrease considerably. Patients with cancers that produce vasopressin ectopically may be in the habit of drinking a customary amount of fluid before the tumor developed; if the same fluid intake is continued after the ectopic vasopressin is present, SIADH may develop even before the cancer is diagnosed.

Any disorder of the lungs, including those requiring respirator care, can cause the release of vasopressin mediated by the volume receptor in the right atrium. Thus, the commonly prescribed increased fluids in pneumonia can precipitate an episode of SIADH. Most neurologic conditions, including meningitis, tumors, the postsurgical condition, and trauma, can increase vasopressin secretion; these potential complications are well recognized and account for the usual orders for reduced fluid administration in neurologic disease. After any surgery there is increased vasopressin secretion, and the patient is susceptible to SIADH; thus the orders to "push fluids" after surgery may precipitate an episode of SIADH. Any condition causing nausea and emesis, including carcinomatosis or the administration of chemotherapy, can increase vasopressin secretion. Further, drugs often used in cancer therapy, such as vancomycin, vincristine, and cytoxan, have their own actions of increasing vasopressin secretion in addition to their tendency to cause nausea. Many types of cancers produce vasopressin in an ectopic hormone secreting syndrome so that a patient with cancer may be susceptible to SIADH from the cancer, from the nausea of the cancer therapy, and from the chemotherapeutic agent itself!

Diagnosis of SIADH

Not all episodes of *hyponatremia* are due to SIADH. The most frequent cause of hyponatremia in pediatrics is fluid overload with hypotonic fluids while on intravenous therapy under a physician's care. Congestive heart failure and the oliguric phase of acute renal failure may lead to hyponatremia. Other conditions lead to low sodium measured on laboratory instruments due to osmotically active substances in the serum; in hyperglycemia (an elevation of atrial naturetic factor causes some real hyponatremia in some cases of diabetic ketoacidosis), hyperlipidemia, and hyperproteinemia (such as in multiple myelosis), there is asymptomatic pseudohyponatremia.

The Treatment of SIADH

The treatment of SIADH is first and foremost prevention. This is primarily an iatrogenic disease, and monitoring fluid therapy with frequent serum sodium concentrations will eliminate the possibility of severe shifts of sodium. Once the SIADH develops fluid restriction to the minimum possible level is the correct approach. In many cases, maintaining intravenous fluids at a level to keep the intravenous line open is appropriate. With less severe hyponatremia, replacing urine output with an equal amount of intravenous fluid figured every two to four hours is adequate fluid replacement. Because the urine flow is so low in SIADH, the tendency will be to fear for inadequate intravascular volume and to decide to administer boluses of fluid to increase urinary output; if the oliguria is due to dehydration, the boluses are appropriate, but if SIADH has been diagnosed, the boluses will only intensify the SIADH. Careful review of the records, including an accounting of all fluid administered (a balance sheet of intake and output is essential), should clear up the diagnosis.

Other methods are available to break through the SIADH. Lithium and democycline will interfere with ADH action on the kidney, but the side effects inherent in their use eliminates them as viable choices. If hyponatremia is severe and seizures have occurred, lasix may be administered to cause some degree of urination and volume depletion. Replacement of the volume loss with 3% saline will help correct the hyponatremia. This procedure of diuretic and hypertonic fluid administration can cause rapid fluid shifts and a patent intravenous line must be maintained to administer the fluid as necessary.

It should be emphasized that the sodium diuresis characteristic of SIADH is continuous during the active phase of the disorder and sodium administered orally or intravenously will quickly be passed out in the urine. Intravenous hypertonic saline likewise will raise serum sodium only temporarily. The only effective treatment of a seizure caused by hyponatremia is raising the sodium concentration. Administration of 3% saline intravenously has been suggested as being helpful on a very temporary basis, but if seizures are intractable, the combination of lasix and hypertonic saline may be the only answer.

Craniopharyngioma Surgery

A patient with a craniopharyngioma already may have diabetes insipidus before surgery for the condition; if not, when the pituitary stalk is cut, diabetes insipidus may manifest on the operating room table. Following this, in a few days, there often will be unrestrained release of vasopressin as the cut nerve cells degenerate; if the high level of fluid replacement originally necessary for treatment of the diabetes insipidus is continued during the vasopressin secretion phase, a full-blown SIADH picture will develop. During the following days a third phase of permanent diabetes insipidus or, in lucky patients where the cut is low on the pituitary stalk, normal vasopressin secretion will develop. It is imperative that fluid output be monitored carefully so that intake is matched to output and fluid overloading does not occur.

Suggested Readings

Bie P: Osmoreceptors, vasopressin and control of renal water excretion. Physiol Rev 1980;60:1961

Bode HH, Crawford JD: Nephrogenic diabetes insipidus in North America; the Hopewell hypotheses. N Engl J Med 1969;280:750

Crawford JD, Kennedy GC: Chlorothiazide in diabetes insipidus. Nature (London) 1959;183:891

Fitzsimons JT: The physiological basis of thirst. Kidney Int 1976;10:3

Freidman AL, Segal WE: Antidiuretic hormone excess. J Pediatr 1979;94:521

Hollinshead WH: The interphase of diabetes insipidus. Proc Mayo Clin 1964;39:92

Rascher W, Tulassay T, Lang RE: Atrial natriuretic peptide in plasma of volume-overloaded children with chronic renal failure. Lancet 1985;2:303

Robertson GL, Berl T: Pathophysiology of water metabolism In: The Kidney. Bremer BM, Rector FC Jr (editors). Philadelphia: Saunders, 1986

Robinson AG: DDAVP in the treatment of central diabetes insipidus. N Engl J Med 1976;294:507

Schwartz WB, Bennet W, Curelop S, et al: A syndrome of renal sodium loss and hyponatremia, probably resulting from inappropriate secretion of antidiuretic hormone. Am J Med 1957;23:529

Chapter 6

Thyroid Gland

Thyroid disease is common in pediatric practice. Although many cases are straightforward, confusion will arise in others. For example, 1 in 10,000 children will have decreased thyroid binding globulin and therefore low total thyroxine (T4) concentrations; no therapy is indicated, but many patients are treated incorrectly with thyroxine. Transient abnormalities of neonatal thyroid function are being recognized increasingly and may be confused with permanent hypothyroidism in regard to therapy and prognosis.

NORMAL THYROID PHYSIOLOGY

Thyroxine is synthesized by the following sequential steps: a) *trapping* of plasma iodide by the thyroid follicular cell; b) *oxidation* of iodide to iodine; c) *organification* of the tyrosine molecules (which are attached to the thyroglobulin molecule) by the addition of one iodine at the 3 position (causing the formation of monoiodotyrosine [MIT]) or two iodines at the 3 and 5 positions (forming diiodotyrosine [DIT]); d) the *coupling* of DIT with DIT to form 3,5,3,5' tetraiodothryronine *(T4)* or one DIT with one MIT to produce 3,5,3' triiodothyronine *(T3)*.

Although both T4 and T3 are released from the thyroid gland, most of the circulating T3 is derived from *peripheral deiodination* of the ß-ring of T4. Reverse T3 (RT3) or 3,3',5' triiodothyronine is a metabolically inert product of the peripheral deiodination of the α-ring of T4.

While the free hormone is the active product, circulating T4 is predominantly bound by serum proteins; 75% is bound to *thyroid binding globulin (TBG)*, 20% to *thyroxine binding pre-albumin (TBPA)*, and 5% to albumin with only 0.20 to 0.06% present in the circulation as *free thyroxine (FT4)*; less than 1% of T_3 circulates as *free T_3 (FT3)*. Present theory holds that free T_3 is the metabolically active form of thyroid hormone and that protein-bound T_3 and T_4 may be considered reservoirs of hormone in equilibrium with the metabolically active free hormone.

The thyroid gland is regulated by the hypothalamus and the pituitary gland. Hypothalamic *thyrotropin releasing hormone (TRF)* is released from the median eminence into the pituitary portal circulation and stimulates the pituitary gland to release *thyrotropin stimulating hormone (TSH)* into the general circulation, whereby it reaches the thyroid gland and stimulates the production and release of thyroid hormones. In the absence of adequate thyroid hormone (*primary hypothyroidism*), TSH rises to very high levels, whereas in the presence of autonomous and excessive production or administration of thyroid hormone, TSH is suppressed.

Laboratory Evaluation of Thyroid Function

Radioimmunoassay of *total T_4 and T_3* and TSH are now generally available. Interpretation of total serum T_4 or T_3 must include simultaneous determination of endogenous protein binding of T_4 and T_3 unless a method is used to measure directly the free hormone. Free T_4 (FT4) and free T_3 (FT3) methods recently have become widely available and are becoming the first choice of a screening test for thyroid dysfunction.

Direct measurement of TBG by RIA is available, but most laboratories still offer an indirect indication of protein binding, such as the resin T_3 uptake (RT3U). The values reported in the RT3U are *inversely proportional to available protein binding sites* in a patient's serum sample. One commonly used method to correct the T_4 for protein binding is to multiply the T_4 by the RT3U with the result called the *free thyroxine index (FTI)*, or the *T7*. Thus, with decreased TBG the total T_4 and T_3 will be low, the RT3U will be high, and the T_4I will be normal. In true hypothyroidism the T_4 will be low and with reduced T_4 the protein binding sites will be more available, thereby lowering the RT3U as well; the FTI will be low. In TBG excess, T_4 and T_3 will be high, but with increased protein binding sites, the RT3U will be low and the resulting T_4I will be normal. In true hyperthyroidism, the T_4 will be high, causing decreased available thyroid binding sites so that the RT3U also will be elevated; as a result of high T_4 and RT3U, the FTI will be high. As a rule of thumb if the T_4 varies from normal and the RT3U varies in the opposite direction, the patient likely will be euthyroid with an abnormality of thyroid binding protein; if the T_4 deviates from normal and the RT3U varies in the same direction, there is likelihood that there is a disorder of thyroid function present. Thus, every patient with a low T_4 is not hypothyroid and does not necessarily require therapy, just as every patient with a high T_4 does not have hyperthyroidism.

Normally, TSH is less than 5 to 7 mIU/ml (depending upon the laboratory standards) so that there is no effective difference between a normal value and a "low" value. New *ultrasensitive TSH assays* are becoming widely available to measure TSH accurately down to 0.5 mIU/ml. Thus a patient with Graves disease will have a value <0.5 mIU/ml and a normal patient will have a value between 0.5 and 5 mIU/ml. In primary hypothyroidism or compensated hypothyroidism, TSH is elevated; in secondary (pituitary defect lacking TSH production) or tertiary (hypothalamic derived due to lack of TRF production) hypothyroidism, the TSH is normally low. The combination of FTI and TSH determination should allow the physician to be able to distinguish between cases of primary hypothyroidism as opposed to secondary or tertiary hypothyroidism. To differentiate between secondary hypothyroidism and tertiary hypothyroidism, however, requires a dynamic TRF test. A dose of 200 µg of TRF is given intravenously and TSH measured at 0, 10, 15, 30, 60, 90, 120, and 180 minutes. A normal response is a rise in TSH to at least 10mIU/ml after about 15 minutes; in secondary hypothyroidism, there will be no rise in TSH, and in tertiary hypothyroidism the rise will be delayed until 60 to 120 minutes and the TSH may continue to rise during the 180 minute period. The TRF test is also useful in the diagnosis of hyperthyroidism, as there will be no rise in TSH with the autonomous thyroxine secretion characteristic of Graves disease.

Thyroid scanning and *radioactive iodine uptake* have a limited role in pediatric diagnosis. Imaging of a thyroid gland is essential for diagnosis in the presence of nodules of the thyroid gland (to determine if they are functional or "cold" and therefore nonfunctional) or for the localization of an ectopic thyroid gland. However, in a clear case of Hashimoto thyroiditis or Graves disease, little is added by a thyroid scan, although they often have been (I believe uselessly) performed in children. The scanning of a neonate or infant presents particular problems; the radioactive trace, which is administered orally, may be spit up by the infant and leave tracts on the skin, falsely suggesting thyroid tissue. Further, a neonate with primary hypothyroidism may have no detectable gland on scan just after birth, but after months to years a normal gland may be detected; in several cases, this has been traced to the transient presence of *thyroid binding inhibitory immunoglobulin (TBII)* in the neonatal circulation that was passed from the mother (who may herself have symptomatic autoimmune thyroid disease) to the fetus. Other cases of *transient hypothyroidism* are due to the use of iodine containing cleaning compounds on the skin of the neonate. A *congenital iodine trapping defect* also will lead to a lack of thyroidal iodine uptake that in this case is not reversible. The demonstration of an ectopic gland in a neonate, however, is good evidence that the child has a permanent defect. In the differential diagnosis of goiter, a *perchlorate discharge test* may be used in which a thyroid uptake is determined and then repeated with the administration of potassium perchlorate, which causes the discharge of nonorganified iodine; if the turnover of iodine is much higher with perchlorate than without, an enzyme deficiency causing an organification defect is present. An important consideration of performing thyroid uptake determinations is to measure the uptake early, such as at four to six hours as well as at 24 hours, because a quick turnover of radioactive iodine, as may occur in Graves disease, may lead to a low uptake at 24 hours but a very high uptake at four to six hours. Scanning is done with ^{123}I or technetium ^{99}m pertechnetate.

Ultrasonographic scanning of the thyroid gland is useful to differentiate cystic from solid masses and the relationship of the mass to neck structures. If a mass is solid, it is more likely to be carcinoma than if it is cystic, and recent studies suggest improved accuracy in the diagnosis of thyroid carcinoma by ultrasonography. Ultrasonography can also be used to guide a biopsy needle, should this be considered advisable in a given case.

DISORDERS OF THE THYROID GLAND

Goiter

An enlargement of the thyroid gland is known as a *goiter* whether the patient is euthyroid, hypothyroid, or hyperthyroid. There is no such condition as "physiologic goiter of adolescence"; recent data suggests that the poorly defined goiters (*colloid goiters*) that may occur at puberty may involve a thyroid antibody. A goiter may be large enough to be noticed by the patient or parent or may be noted on routine examination or during an investigation of symptoms. Palpation usually is best accomplished with the examiner's fingers directed anteriorly around the neck while the examiner stands behind the patient. If the patient swallows water during the examination, the mobile nature of the thyroid gland may be appreciated as it rises and falls on swallowing. *Hashimoto thyroiditis* may be accompanied by a midline, pea-sized *Delphian node* located 0.5 to 1 cm above the isthmus; the Delphian node does not move with swallowing. The margins of the goiter should be noted distinct from the neighboring sternocleidomastoid muscle, and measurement should be recorded; I find it best to record the horizontal distance of each lobe, the vertical distance of each lobe, and the height of the isthmus. Some observers find it useful to trace the outline of the gland on a piece of tissue paper and to include it in the patient's record for future comparison. It is difficult to estimate the weight of the thyroid gland in children as is done in adult patients, but an estimation of the number of times the gland appears to be increased over normal size can be accomplished more easily.

The thyroid functional status is determined after it has been ascertained that the patient has a goiter. Most goiters in early childhood or infancy will be diagnosed by the newborn screening programs and will be due to maternal ingestion of goitrogen or an inborn error of thyroid biosynthesis. The majority of goiters in the late childhood-adolescent years will be due to euthyroid or hypothyroid Hashimoto thyroiditis followed by a lower incidence of Graves disease. There will remain a minority of indeterminate goiters of mild degree that may persist for years; these may be colloid goiters, a diagnosis that is established only after all other diagnoses are eliminated. Colloid goiter is not accompanied by an elevation in serum antimicrosomal or antithyroglobulin antibody levels or, usually, an alteration in thyroid function from normal.

A *solitary nodule* in childhood is unusual and worthy of careful attention. A thyroid scan is indicated to determine whether the nodule is hot and functional, or cold and nonfunctional. A *cold nodule* is particularly worrisome, as it may indicate neoplasia (see below). A palpable nodule that is indistinguishable from the rest of the gland on thyroid scan may be followed without surgical intervention; thyroxine therapy may cause it to shrink.

Hypothyroidism

Neonatal Hypothyroidism

The detection and treatment of neonates with hypothyroidism should be considered as a pediatric emergency. If therapy is not begun soon after birth, mental retardation will result. *Neonatal hypothyroidism* is a relatively common disorder, with an incidence close to 1 in 4000 live births. Routine *neonatal screening* has been instituted in most states and countries due to the difficulty in making the diagnosis early enough on clinical grounds alone. Heelstick samples of blood are collected on a filter paper and sent to a centralized laboratory, where blood is eluted from the paper and analyzed for concentration of T_4. If the value is low for the laboratory runs for the day, a TSH is performed. If the T_4 is low and the TSH is high, a diagnosis of presumptive primary hypothyroidism is made; if the T_4 is low and the TSH is also low, the patient may be referred for further evaluation to rule out secondary or tertiary hypothyroidism.

It is important to view the normal developmental physiology of the fetus and newborn in order to understand the pitfalls of the neonatal screening program. By 10 to 11 weeks of gestation, the human thyroid gland shows follicular organization and demonstrates iodine concentrating ability. By this time, TRF is demonstrable in the fetal hypothalamus, and TSH is found in the fetal pituitary and circulation. The pituitary hypothalamic portal system is developing around this time and is mostly mature by 30 weeks' gestation. Thus, most of the components of thyroid physiology are in place by the second half of gestation.

Fetal serum concentration of the thyroid hormones reflect this maturation, as none of the thyroid hormones or TSH cross the placenta in appreciable amounts. Serum TSH rises at about 20 weeks of gestation, as TRF is able to reach the pituitary gland, and T_4 rises as a result. In the fetus the vast majority of T_4 is α-ring deiodinated, leading to the formation of RT_3 in parallel with concentrations of T_4. Late in gestation, the ß-ring deiodination increases, and T_3 finally begins to rise as well. At term, then, fetal TSH and T_4 are slightly higher than normal adult concentrations, fetal serum RT_3 is markedly higher than in the adult, and fetal serum T_3 is considerably lower. TBG and other thyroid binding proteins rise with advancing gestation as do other serum proteins.

After delivery, TSH quickly rises and peaks at 30 minutes, T_4 is secreted in response and peaks at 24 to 72 hours, T_3 exhibits a primary rise in the hours after birth due to increased ß-ring deiodination of T_4 and exhibits a secondary rise at 24 to 72 hours; RT_3 falls after birth due to the switch from α-ring deiodination to ß-ring deiodination; TBG and therefore the RT_3U remain constant with parturition.

A normal term child will have serum T_4 concentrations in the adult hyperthyroid range during the 24 to 72 hours after birth, and a bona fide hypothyroid child will have T_4 either below or in the normal adult range. Healthy premature babies, interrupted before the normal end point of thyroid physiologic development at term, have a lower concentration of the thyroid hormones, and premature babies with respiratory distress syndrome have values lower still. Small-for-gestational-age infants likewise have lower thyroid hormone concentrations than do normal children. Thus, it should be clear that the gestational age of the neonate, the clinical condition, and in fact, the postnatal age are important in the interpretation of neonatal thyroid screening tests. The majority of false positive tests reported from a screening center will be from premature babies or small-for-gestational-age infants with low T_4 concentrations and normally low TSH.

The signs and symptoms of *congenital hypothyroidism* in its classic form include large tongue, coarse facies, umbilical hernia, a combination of lethargy and irritability, poor growth and weight gain, short extremities with a delayed or high upper-to-lower segment ratio, persistently open posterior fontanel, large anterior fontanel, and coarse voice. Further, pericardial edema can be noted on ultrasound study in infants untreated for a prolonged time. However, these signs and symptoms take weeks to months to develop, and if suspicion of congenital hypothyroidism was to be triggered by physical stigmata, the majority of patients would have to wait until irreversible mental changes already were established. It is true that features such as prolonged gestation with large birth weight, persistent jaundice, temperature instability, lag in the time of the initial stool to more than 20 hours after birth, edema, and hypoactivity and poor feeding can be seen in such patients in the neonatal period, but these are signs of other diseases as well and may not strongly suggest the diagnosis to the physician.

Thus, neonatal screening programs were established to diagnose patients uniformly before definitive symptoms occur. The signs and symptoms of congenital hypothyroidism must be remembered because the statewide screening programs are not infallible, and a few patients have missed screening because of home birth, early discharge from the hospital, long stay in the neonatal intensive care unit, transfer between hospitals, or because of lost samples. If a suspicion exists about a patient, rather than waiting for the neonatal screening result, a clinical T_4 and TSH determination can be requested, and the results, in some cases, may be available sooner than from the screening program.

The etiology of congenital hypothyroidism is usually *athyreosis, hypoplasia of the thyroid gland,* or a lack of descent of the thyroid gland from its initial site of formation at the back of the tongue at the foramen cecum to its normal mature location (*thyroid ectopy* or *"cryptothyroidism"*). A thyroid scan will demonstrate ectopy, but initial athyreosis or hypoplasia on scan may be due to blocking antibodies, as mentioned above, and may falsely suggest a permanent anatomic abnormality when in fact a transient condition is present.

Biochemical abnormalities of the thyroid gland are usually hereditary and often involve the appearance of a goiter. Possibilities include *dyshormonogenesis,* such as *peroxidase defects (organification defects), iodotyrosine deiodinase defect,* and *thyroglobulin defects* (causing lack of coupling of MIT and DIT). A *defect in TSH receptors* and a *defect in the transport of iodine* into the gland have been described and do not lead to goiter. Several families are described with *peripheral resistance to thyroid hormone;* thyroid hormone and TSH concentrations are high, but the patients are clinically euthyroid but may have deaf-mutism, skeletal abnormalities, and goiter.

Congenital hypopituitarism may include *secondary or tertiary hypothyroidism* as a feature, but there will be other pituitary hormone deficiencies present as well. Rarely (<1:100,000 live births), *isolated TSH deficiency* is seen.

External agents can cause congenital hypothyroidism when they are administered to the mother. *Radioactive iodine* mistakenly given to a pregnant woman with Graves disease (possibly because she denied being pregnant) will immediately cross the placenta and damage the developing gland. *Propylthiouracil (PTU)* given to a pregnant woman with hyperthyroidism also will cross the placenta and can cause profound hypothyroidism; when the PTU is cleared postpartum, the baby will recover from the suppression and hypo-thyroidism, and the thyroid-stimulating immunoglobulin that was passed from the mother will begin to exert its effect, causing transient hyperthyroidism. Paradoxically, *excessive iodine* given to the mother can suppress thyroid gland formation just as a *deficiency of iodine* can.

There are several situations where thyroid binding proteins are altered and thereby alter the serum T_4 and T_3 concentration. *Decreased thyroid binding globulin,* or *TBG deficiency,* occurs in 1:10000 live births in a sex-linked pattern. The serum T_4 and T_3 are decreased, and the child will be picked up by the newborn screening program. *Familial dysalbuminemic hyperthyroxinemia (FDH)* leads to increased T_4 but a normal serum T_3; the free form of both hormones are normal, and the patient is asymptomatic.

With the receipt of a screening test suggesting congenital hypothyroidism, another set of serum samples for confirmatory T_4 and TSH should be drawn, as the screening test is, as stated, simply a screening test requiring proof. If the initial T_4 was very low and the TSH was quite high, treatment with synthetic T_4 may be started while awaiting the results of the confirmatory tests. The decision of whether to perform a thyroid scan is controversial due to the false positives as noted above; in the absence of a goiter or a strikingly low T_4 and high TSH, we do not perform them. A *bone age deter-mination* of the knee and foot is quite useful: the distal femoral epiphysis calcifies at 36 weeks of gestation, the proximal tibial at 38 weeks, and the cuboid at term. Thus, a bone age can be determined at the time of receipt of the screening results and the finding of delayed bone age may strengthen the impression of congenital hypothyroidism. Patients with congenital hypothyroidism may have epiphyseal dysgenesis or irregular multifocal calcification on x-ray after the epiphyses do appear.

Transient hyperthyrotropinemia has been described in which a child will have perfectly normal T_4 concentrations for age but a slightly elevated TSH (often in the range of 20 to 30 mIU/ml.) The natural history of such patients is a decrease in the TSH concentrations to normal by one to two years of age in the absence of treatment. Children with laboratory values characteristic of transient hyperthyrotropinemia should be watched for evidence of decreasing thyroid function in case they have an ectopic or hypoplastic thyroid gland that decompensates with time. Such patients may maintain a normal T_4 concentration at the time of the newborn screening at the expense of an elevated TSH.

Treatment of congenital hypothyroidism should begin when the diagnosis is established; as mentioned above, confirmatory tests beyond the neonatal screening tests must be obtained. In those cases where the screening results show an extremely low T_4 and high TSH, treatment can be started before the confirmatory results are available, as it will be most unlikely that a mistake in diagnosis has occurred. Presently, recommended dosage of synthetic thyroxine is 10 μg/kg for the newborn (a dose of 25 μg is the usual daily dose in term newborns) and 2 to 5 μg/kg per day after one year of age with an eventual total dose of 100 to 150 μg at the maximum in a teenager. Thyroxine is most widely available in tablets and is crushed and administered in a small amount of formula or applesauce. Liquid thyroxine is available for parenteral use but is quite expensive; it has been used for patients who are unable to take medications orally. It is becoming more common to test patients at three years of age to see if they have permanent hypothyroidism or one of the transient defects; in only those patients that have reliable families and can be counted upon to return for followup, thyroxine can be discontinued for two to four weeks with T_4 and TSH measured at tow and four weeks to determine function. Most brain growth is completed at three years, but it is not advisable to leave a child off thyroxine for any longer interval if function appears impaired.

Neonates with congenital hypothyroidism may have elevated TSH concentrations for months or even years after the onset of therapy due to a persistent abnormality of feedback suppression; attempting to suppress these TSH concentrations will lead to excessive thyroxine dosage. Thus, the goal of therapy should be to maintain a normal serum thyroxine concentration for age rather than to suppress the TSH to normal values for age. Overtreatment with thyroxine will cause advancement of the bone age and can lead to craniosynostosis. Further, the administration of normal dosages of thyroxine to infants with congenital hypothyroidism that are untreated for a period of months may cause the onset of congestive heart failure due to the rapid mobilization of fluid accumulated during the myxedematous state; in such children, with late onset of therapy, it is preferable to work up to the full dose over a period of 7 to 14 days.

Patients treated early and appropriately with thyroxine are likely to have normal intelligence, according to recent follow-up studies; there may be some subtle hearing or motor dysfunction in these children. There is evidence that if the bone age is delayed at the time of institution of therapy in the infant, the intellectual function may be more impaired than if the bone age is normal; this suggests that a patient with more profound hypothyroidism as reflected in the delay in skeletal maturation will suffer intrauterine brain damage. Further, there are cases on record where even therapy begun in the first week of life does not eliminate severe intellectual impairment. Nonetheless, the institution of neonatal thyroid screening and neonatal treatment has markedly decreased the morbidity of this common condition.

Acquired Hypothyroidism

Childhood hypothyroidism starting after two years of age does not carry the risk of permanent mental retardation as does neonatal hypothyroidism, but temporary behavior changes are frequent. Remarkably, children with *acquired hypothyroidism* may have improved grades due to their longer attention span, whereas with treatment their reduced attention span causes their grades to fall! Mild congenital abnormalities, such as an ectopic thyroid gland, may first manifest in the childhood period, although most will have been diagnosed by moderate elevations of the TSH level in the newborn screening programs. Further, the addition of iodine to food in the United States has effectively eliminated endemic iodine deficient goiter in this country.

Hashimoto, or chronic lymphocytic thyroiditis, is responsible for the majority of cases of acquired hypothyroidism. This autoimmune disorder is found in a continuum with Graves disease, and both disorders may coexist or one may be followed by the other. Both disorders occur frequently in a family pattern. In Hashimoto thyroiditis, a genetic disposition leads to the formation of unsuppressed clones of thymus dependent lymphocytes directed against the thyroid gland, causing lymphocytic infiltration of the gland. B-lymphocytes, either through interaction with T-lymphocytes or because of stimulation linked to the damaged thyroid cells, produce antithyroid antibodies that are so characteristic of the disorder. Hashimoto thyroiditis frequently is associated with diabetes mellitus and Turner syndrome so that patients with either condition should undergo surveillance for the development of this condition. Clinical characteristics include goiter, a Delphian node (a pea-sized, centrally located lymph node just above the thyroid gland), minimally to severely elevated TSH concentrations, a positive titer of *antimicrosomal antibodies* or *antithyroglobulin antibodies,* and frequently a family history of thyroid disease.

Normal to slightly elevated TSH concentrations with normal T_4I or free T_4 indicates *euthyroid goiter* or *compensated hypothyroidism.* Elevated TSH and decreased free T_3 or free T_4 indicates obvious primary hypothyroidism. If the TSH is elevated, the treatment is clear: the administration of thyroxine until the TSH is suppressed to normal and the serum T_4 is normal. If the TSH is not elevated and the goiter is minimal, the patient may be watched for further deterioration in thyroid function. If the goiter is cosmetically noticeable, thyroxine may be given for a period of three months to see if the goiter can be shrunk; if the small goiter does not change, thyroxine may be stopped and the patient followed for a time when the thyroxine may be more necessary.

There are other causes for acquired hypothyroidism besides Hashimoto thyroiditis. A *thyroglossal duct cyst* in the midline of the neck may contain the complete complement of functioning thyroid tissue available to the patient; if any midline congenital defect is removed surgically, the patient must be followed for the development of hypothyroidism, or the patient should have a thyroid scan to confirm the presence of remaining thyroid tissue. Some children are born with only one lobe of thyroid gland, usually the left. This tissue may undergo compensatory hypertrophy and it has the usual chance of developing Hashimoto thyroiditis, causing hypothyroidism.

Acquired hypothyroidism is treated with thyroxine in a dose of approximately 3-5 μg/kg to a maximum of 100-150 μg. Unlike neonates with congenital hypothyroidism, older children can have their dose titrated to suppress the TSH to normal.

Abnormalities of thyroid binding proteins may be congenital, but also may be acquired. Thus, increased TBG binding of thyroid hormones occurs with estrogen treatment or pregnancy or in the presence of an inherited condition; decreased TBG binding of thyroid hormones occurs with androgen therapy, protein-losing conditions, dilantin therapy and an X-linked genetic condition.

Hyperthyroidism

Hyperthyroidism, or Graves disease, is also an autoimmune disease and, as noted, may coexist with Hashimoto thyroiditis. *Thyroid stimulatory IgG (TSI) antibodies* are formed and directed toward the

TSH receptor, leading to autonomous thyroid function and hyperthyroidism. T_3 is produced more efficiently than in the normal state and both T_4 and T_3 exceed the TBG capacity so that free T_4 and free T_3 rise. In some cases, the T_4 is normal but the T_3 is elevated; in the diagnosis of hyperthyroidism, both should be measured. Increased autonomic tone can cause lid retraction and "stare." Exophthalmos may occur due to infiltration of glycoprotein in the posterior of the orbit. Pretibial myxedema is found in some patients. Weakness, increased pulse, emotional lability to the point of apparent psychiatric disease, hyperactivity, and lack of attention span, weight loss, and diarrhea are characteristic findings.

Thyroid storm consists of acute onset of hyperthermia and tachycardia in a patient with underlying hyperthyroidism; it is far rarer in childhood than in the adult patient. Precipitating factors are surgery, infection, and diabetic ketoacidosis. Symptoms include high fever, sweating, tachycardia, and reduced mental state ranging from confusion to coma. Immediate therapy is indicated for this severe condition.

Propranolol (5 to 10 mg every six hours as a starting dose) can control some symptoms of thyroid storm. Propranolol can be given intravenously at a dose of 0.1 mg/kg up to a total of 5 mg, but an intra-atrial pacing catheter is a necessary precaution. Dexamethasone in a dose of 1 to 2 mg every 6 hours can lower serum T_3. Intravenous NaI in a dose of 1 to 2 grams per day may decrease the release of thyroid hormone from the thyroid gland; Lugol's solution can be given orally if the patient is conscious. A cooling blanket can help control the hyperpyrexia. Propylthiouracil will not take effect for several days, but to plan for the possibly extended course of the disorder, 200 to 300 mg can be given every six hours by slurry, if necessary. Fluid management must be watched and, if tachycardia causes heart failure, digitalis may be necessary.

Laboratory findings in hyperthyroidism are elevated T_4 and T_3 (both in either the total or free determination) with non-detectable TSH, positive thyroid stimulating immunoglobulin titer, and often low positive titers of antithyroglobulin and antimicrosomal antibodies; if the titers of antimicrosomal and antithyroglobulin antibodies are very elevated, the patient may have the combination of Graves disease and Hashimoto thyroiditis. It is usually not necessary to perform a thyroid scan if the constellation of symptoms are classic. A complete blood count is useful to detect any changes in the white blood cell count due to the hyperthyroid state; the white blood cell count may be decreased in hyperthyroidism and may be decreased further by medical therapy for hyperthyroidism. I suggest an ANA and SMA20 be determined if propylthiouracil is to be invoked as treatment to ensure that no abnormalities are present before medication is given.

There are three possible types of *treatment for hyperthyroidism: medication, radiation therapy,* and *surgery.* Propylthiouracil (PTU) or methimazole are the medical therapies available in the United States; in Europe, carbamazole is also available. PTU blocks organification and decreases T_4 to T_3 conversion and may inhibit the formation of the offending IgG, whereas methimazole only demonstrates the first activity. PTU is given in does of 150 to 450 mg/day divided into doses given every eight hours. The aim is to cause a sufficient block to cause hypothyroidism and then to add replacement thyroxin to cause a euthyroid state. The patient is followed for shrinkage of the gland, an essential finding if remission is to be expected. There is an incidence of remission of 25% every two years that patients are followed with medical therapy: thus, after 11 years of therapy, 75% of patients in the series achieved remission. Serious side effects of PTU or methimazole are rare but can be life threatening. Lupus-like syndromes, rashes, granulocytopenia or agranulocytosis, and hepatitis possibly leading to cirrhosis can occur in a usually reversible fashion and are generally idiosyncratic, occurring early in the course of therapy. These drugs should be stopped if such side effects are found and alternative methods of therapy used. Lack of compliance, unfortunately a common condition in this age group, is also an indication for surgical or radioiodine therapy.

Propranolol (5 to 10 mg every six hours as a starting dose) can control symptoms of hyperthyroidism and is useful in short-term situations such as in preparation for surgery or in the face of thyroid storm; side effects of propranolol upon respiratory or circulatory function are possible. Studies have shown propranolol to be helpful for long-term management in adults, but it has not generally been used as such in children.

Subtotal thyroidectomy is an alternative therapy. An experienced thyroid surgeon should perform the operation so that complications will be unlikely. Recurrent laryngeal nerve paralysis is an unusual but possible complication. Hypocalcemia can follow thyroidectomy transiently due to postoperative edema of the parathyroid glands, or permanently if the parathyroid glands are removed with the thyroid tissue. Preparation for surgery involves the use of medical management to control the hyperthyroid state followed by supersaturated iodine solution (Lugol's, eight drops per day) for the ten days prior to surgery. The iodine will harden the gland and reduce the blood supply to the gland. Iodine has only a temporary effect in suppressing thyroxine secretion from the hyperthyroid gland; escape usually will occur after two to four weeks. Although the surgeon may be able to remove the optimal amount of tissue to allow euthyroid function after surgery, more often the patient will be hypothyroid after surgery. By ten years after surgery, almost all patients will be hypothyroid due to continued scarring and reduced function of the remaining thyroid tissue.

Radioactive iodine (^{131}I) therapy has been used in hyperthyroidism for more than 40 years and has proved safe in studies of children and adolescents so treated and of their subsequent offspring. However, although there is no documentation of statistically increased risk, some consider it ill-advised to administer radioactive iodine to children for a potentially reversible condition; it has been suggested that the younger the child receives the radioactive iodine, the more likely the development of carcinoma and that there is yet inadequate data to state that this form of therapy is safe in childhood. Further, one dose of radioactive iodine may not cure the patient, and another dose may be necessary. After the treatment, some patients may be euthyroid, but as in surgical treatment, by ten years post-therapy almost all will be hypothyroid due to continued scarring of the gland.

Neonates can have bona fide Graves disease, but most newborns with hyperthyroidism have acquired it from transplacentally acquired thyroid stimulating immunoglobulin (TSI). As the mother is usually on therapy with PTU, the child will have been exposed to levels of PTU, which does freely cross the placenta. The child may be born profoundly hypothyroid and in fact suffer severe respiratory insufficiency due to pressure on the trachea exerted by the goiter caused by PTU during fetal life. The hypothyroid phase often will trigger the statewide screening program to report the child as a presumptive positive hypothyroid child with a low T_4 and a high TSH. After 3 to 6 days, as the PTU leaves the circulation, the child will bear the brunt of the TSI effect and develop nervousness, diarrhea, shakiness, and tachycardia. The infant can receive Lugol's solution of iodine to suppress thyroid hormone output, propranolol to counter the effects of hyperthyroidism, or PTU if the condition seems severe and may last for several months.

Neoplasms

Carcinomas of the thyroid gland are rare in childhood, but certain historic features increase the likelihood of a thyroid mass being malignant. A history of prior irradiation of the thyroid gland (e.g., for acne, enlarged thymus, or ringworm) is significant, and if the irradiation was done for the therapy of another cancer (e.g., at the time of bone marrow transplant), the risk is higher. However, the local radiation used for the treatment of Graves disease appears not to be a etiology for thyroid carcinoma, as it kills the thyroid follicular cells as it controls the Graves disease.

A single firm nodule is more ominous than multiple nodular goiter. Lack of concentration of ^{123}I on thyroid scan (a *cold nodule)* increases the likelihood of carcinoma more than does a functioning nodule (*warm* or *hot nodule).* Ultrasonographic evidence that the nodule is a cyst makes it less likely to be malignant, but carcinomas have been found in the walls of thyroid cysts. The presence of anterior cervical lymph nodes, metastases on chest x-ray, or hoarseness all make the likelihood greater that the single thyroid nodule is malignant. A patient with a family or personal history of multiple endocrine neoplasia syndrome has a great likelihood of having medullary carcinoma of the thyroid gland.

The steps involved in the diagnosis of a solitary nodule are either *needle biopsy* or *open surgical biopsy.* Needle biopsy is safe and has a low level of false negative results, but the experience of the local pathologists in performing and reading needle biopsy specimens is important in making the choice. Even if a needle biopsy suggests a benign diagnosis, if the nodule fails to shrink on suppressive thyroxine therapy over the ensuing months, it may require open excisional biopsy as well. In the absence of experienced clinical help in the procedure of needle biopsy or in a situation heavily suggestive of a malignant diagnosis, open-needle biopsy seems best.

Painful Thyroid Glands

Tenderness of the thyroid gland may indicate a viral infection (*subacute thyroiditis)* or a bacterial infection (*suppurative thyroiditis).* Either of these conditions will be accompanied by an elevated sedimentation rate. Unless an abscess is palpable or visible on ultrasound exam, a needle biopsy for culture may be necessary to differentiate between the two. Bacterial infections are treated with appropriate antibiotics and viral infections with pain medications.

Suggested Readings

Bilanuik LT, Moshang T, Cara J, et al: Pituitary enlargement mimicking pituitary tumor. J Neurosurg 1985;63:39

Bright GM, Robert M, Blizzard RD, Kaiser DL, Clark WL: Organ specific autoantibodies in children with common endocrine diseases. J Pediatr 1982;100:8

Burman KD, Baker JR: Immunomechanisms in Graves disease. Endocrinol Rev 1985;6:183

Cooper DS: Antithyroid drugs. N Engl J Med 1984;311:1353

Emerson CH, Braverman LE: Thyroid irradiation-one view. N Engl J Med 1980;303:217

Fisher DA, Sack J, Oddie TH, et al: Serum T_4 TBG T_3 uptake T_3 reverse T_3 TSH concentrations in children 1 to 15 years of age. J Clin Endocrinol Metab 1977;45:191

Fisher DA, Klein AH: Thyroid development and disorders of thyroid function in the newborn. N Engl J Med 1981;304:702

Glorieux J, Dussault JH, Morissete, et al: Follow-up at ages 5 and 7 years on mental development in children with hypothyroidism detected by Quebec Screening Program. J Pediatr 1985;107:913

Lippe BM, Landow EM, Kaplan SA: Hyperthyroidism in children treated with long-term medical therapy: Twenty-five percent remission every two years. J Clin Endocrinol Metab 1987;64:1241

Maenpaa J, Raatrika M, Rasanen J, et al: Natural course of juvenile autoimmune thyroiditis. J Epidemiol 1985;107:898

New England Congenital Hypothyroidism Collaborative: Neonatal hypothyroidism screening: Status of patients at 6 years.   J Pediatr 1986;107:915

Rallion ML, Dobyns BM, Keating FR, Rall JE, Zyler FH: Occurrence and natural history of chronic lymphocytic thyroiditis in childhood. J Pediatr 1975;86:675

Rovet J, Ehrlich R, Sorbara D: Intellectual outcome in children with fetal hypothyroidism. J Pediatr 1987;110:700

Safa AM, Schumacher OP, Rodriquez-Antunez A: Long-term follow-up results in children and adolescents treated with radioactive iodine (^{131}I) for hyperthyroidism. N Engl J Med 1975;292:167

Wolff J: Congenital goiter with defective iodide transport. Endocrine Rev 1983;4:240

Zucker AR, Chernow B, Fields AI, et al: Thyroid function in critically ill children. J Pediatr 1985;107:552

Chapter 7

Calcium Metabolism

The concentration of calcium in plasma or serum is regulated at between 8.8 and 10 mg/dl by the *vitamin D endocrine system*. In this system, hypocalcemia leads to a decline in ionized calcium concentrations, which stimulates the secretion of *parathyroid hormone* (*PTH*). Newly secreted PTH stimulates the activity of the renal proximal tubule mitochondrial enzyme 1-a-hydroxylase, which converts *25-hydroxyvitamin D* (*25(OH)D*) to *1,25 dihydroxyvitamin D* (*1,25(OH)$_2$D* or *calcitrol*). This 1,25(OH)$_2$D is the most active form of vitamin D detected to date and represents a renal metabolite that acts in the small intestine to increase the active absorption of calcium from the intestinal lumen. 1,25(OH)$_2$D and PTH work together to promote bone resorption at the osteoclastic bone surface, which also releases calcium and phosphate from their bone reservoirs. Enhanced renal tubular calcium reabsorption is another physiologic response to the action of 1,25(OH)$_2$D (see Appendix 7, Table 7-1).

These three sites of action, gut, bone, and distal renal tubule, are removed from the site of 1,25(OH)$_2$D synthesis; thus, 1,25(OH)$_2$D is the hormonal form of vitamin D. When sufficient calcium has been absorbed, resorbed, and reabsorbed to normalize serum calcium values, then PTH secretion falls and 1,25(OH)$_2$D synthesis declines. This feedback regulated scheme represents the vitamin D endocrine system and its response to hypocalcemia. Because vitamin D is activated at one site (the kidney) and moves, via the circulation, bound to a vitamin D binding protein of 52K dalton, to its target sites, vitamin D is no longer a vitamin but rather a hormone. Further, if one conceives that a vitamin is an essential foodstuff that is required in the diet and needed to prevent a deficiency disease, then vitamin D, which has its precursor (7-dehydrochol-esterol) synthesized in the skin and its major circulating form $(1,25(OH)_2D)$ synthesized by hepatocytes and renal tubular cells, no longer fits this definition. Indeed, armed with this understanding of the vitamin D endocrine system, one can appreciate that vitamin D deficiency rickets did not appear as a disorder until the skies of urban areas of northern Europe were blackened by the industrial revolution.

HYPOCALCEMIC DISORDERS

The symptoms of *hypocalcemia* are due to decreased stability of neural membranes. Neuromuscular irritability is manifested by muscle cramps, weakness, lethargy, paresthesias of the extremities, and tetany. Children also can have convulsions and laryngospasm. Three prominent signs indicating hypocalcemia are Chvostek sign, wherein a brisk tap to the facial nerve below the zygomatic arch elicits a twitch at the angle of the mouth; Trousseau sign, where inflating a blood pressure cuff at least 15 mm Hg above the systolic blood pressure results in carpopedal spasms; and the peroneal sign, wherein tapping the peroneal nerve near the lateral tibial prominence leads to plantar flexion. *Tetany* also can appear in hypokalemia, in hypomagnesemia, and with respiratory alkalosis, where the ionized fraction of calcium falls due to enhanced protein binding. Other signs are calcification of the basal ganglia, cataracts, and poor enamel formation of the teeth, particularly if hypocalcemia is present since infancy.

Rickets

Vitamin D deficiency during childhood will result in hypocalcemia, hypophosphatemia, increased serum alkaline phosphatase activity, and secondary hyperparathyroidism with elevated PTH values. Because the concentrations of calcium and phosphate are reduced, chondrocytes in the growth plate of long bones and osteoid, the collagen-contain-ing organic matrix of the bone trabeculum, fail to mineralize normally. This deficiency of mineralization results in the bone lesion called rickets. This lesion appears as undermineralization of the growth plate, an indistinct and ragged metaphysis, and bowing due to the influence of weight bearing on bones lacking their tensile strength. This lesion is apparent by conventional radiographs of the long bones.

Nutritional Rickets

Nutritional rickets does not occur with any frequency in the United States and Canada, as milk is supplemented with 400 IU (10 μg) of vitamin D/liter; most children in Western Europe receive vitamin D in capsule form. Several circumstances result in vitamin D deficient rickets in children throughout the world. First, if children have reasons not to be exposed to the sun, the conversion of 7-dehydrocholesterol to vitamin D_3 will be limited. Children with dark skins living at northern latitudes, wearing heavy robes, or remaining indoors are at particular risk for developing rickets. These include Arabic children, black children in inner cities, and the offspring of parents who are followers of religious sects forbidden to ingest a vegetarian (nondairy-containing) diet, exclusively breastfed, and wear heavy dark robes.

In the United Kingdom and Europe, rickets are found among dark-skinned Asian and Turkish immigrants. Rickets also may occur in retarded, institutionalized children who eschew dairy products and remain indoors. The diagnosis is made by serum chemistry determinations and the finding of a serum 25(OH)D value of under 8 ng/mi, which indicates inadequate vitamin D stores. Normal 25(OH)D is 15 to 60 ng/ml. Treatment of these children with conventional vitamin D at 800 to 2000 IU (20 to 50 μg) daily is usually curative, although additional calcium intake may be required.

Hepatocellular Rickets

Rickets, in conjunction with hepatocellular disorders--biliary atresia, neonatal hepatitis, some hereditary liver disease, and, rarely, cystic fibrosis--occurs by three pathogenic mechanisms. First, malabsorption of ingested vitamin D is common due to a reduction in intraduodenal bile salt concentrations in these children, so this fat soluble vitamin is lost in the stool. Second, hepatic 25-hydroxylation can be reduced in activity. Third, since vitamin D is excreted in bile, the enterohepatic circulation of vitamin D may be interrupted. Of these, the first mechanism appears to be the most relevant. Therapy with 1000 to 2000 IU (25 to 50 μg) daily may heal this form of rickets, but the use of oral 25(OH)D at 25 to 50 μg daily will heal rickets even in children with biliary atresia. In that malabsorption of vitamin D is a major factor in this form of hypocalcemia, phototherapy using ultraviolet light could be used to activate the photocutaneous vitamin D metabolic pathway. The length of sun or ultraviolet light exposure, however, is unclear.

Anticonvulsant Associated Hypocalcemia

Rickets occurring in children receiving anticonvulsant therapy is more common in institutionalized, nonambulatory retarded children. Anticonvulsants, especially phenobarbital and hydantoins, increase the metabolism of 25(OH)D to more inactive, more highly polar metabolites, thereby reducing the supply of the substrate for 1-a-hydroxylase. Perhaps more importantly, these children have diminished intake of dairy products and reduced sunlight exposure. In ambulatory children receiving anticonvulsants, evidence of metabolic bone disease is uncommon. Treatment with 800 IU (20 μg) of vitamin D will assure correction of hypocalcemia and hypophosphatemia in these children, especially if calcium intake is assured.

Rickets of Prematurity

Disorders of bone mineralization are not uncommon in very low birth weight preterm infants. These infants have not benefited from the placental transfer of calcium (150 mg/kg body weight/day) or phosphate (75 mg/kg/day) during the last trimester. The immature intestine cannot efficiently transfer calcium and neither human milk nor cows' milk formulas can match the transfer to the fetus provided by the placenta. Unless the mother has vitamin D deficiency, vitamin D deficiency in these infants is rare, although it should be expected in inner city children. It appears that the peak of 25 hydroxylation activity has not been achieved in these infants due to a generalized hepatic hydroxylation immaturity. However, in general, the serum concentration of 1,25(OH)$_2$D is extremely high, exceeding 120 pg/ml (normal=50 to 80 pg/ml). The stimulus for these high values of 1,25(OH)$_2$D appears to be the hypocalcemia and hypophosphatemia in these infants.

The clinical signs in these infants are hypocalcemia, hypophosphatemia, elevated alkaline phosphatase activity, rib and limb fractures, and rachitic changes at the end of long bones. Multiple fractures are not uncommon. Because mineral deficiency is probably the reason for most cases of rickets, treatment consists of the use of calcium and phosphate supplements in the infant's milk, the use of high-mineral formulas, and additional vitamin D. These infants are extremely difficult to treat if they also have bronchopulmonary dysplasia and are receiving chronic loop diuretic therapy, which promotes hypercalcuria.

Inherited Causes of Rickets

First described by Prader, a rare form of rickets called *Vitamin D dependency rickets* is characterized by a failure of conventional doses of vitamin D to reverse rickets, hypocalcemia, and hypophosphatemia. Patients with this autosomal recessive condition require massive doses of vitamin D (200,000 to 1,000,000 IU daily) to cure the rickets. The levels of 25(OH)D are normal or high, and of 1,25(OH)$_2$D are low, indicating that the enzyme activity of 1-α-hydroxylase is reduced. As evidence to support this mechanism, all the features described can be reversed by physiologic doses (0.5 to 1.0 μg) of 1,25(OH)$_2$D. This disorder also appears at 12 to 16 weeks of age, as would be consistent with a congenital condition.

Some children with vitamin D dependency do not respond to either high dose vitamin D or $1,25(OH)_2D$ at even higher doses. Indeed, in the presence of extremely high levels of $1,25(OH)_2D$ (exceeding 150 pg/ml; normal 15-60 pg/ml), rickets, hypocalcemia, enamel hypoplasia, and signs of secondary hyperparathyroidism are found. A defect in the binding of $1,25(OH)_2D$ to its nuclear receptor best explains these findings. This disorder has been termed *vitamin D dependency rickets, type II*. Some patients with this condition have short stature and total alopecia. These patients can be the offspring of first cousin marriages as it is an autosomal recessive disorder. Treatment of patients with this disorder is difficult, often requiring in excess of 10 μg of $1,25(OH)_2D$ daily.

The most common form of inherited rickets and, indeed, the most prevalent rachitic condition, is *X-linked hypophosphatemic rickets*, or, as it is sometimes called, *vitamin D resistant rickets*. These patients have normocalcemia and hypophosphatemia, with phosphate concentrations insufficient to support mineralization. This condition becomes evident within ages one and two years, with bowing of the lower extremities. Patients do not have tetany, myopathy, a rachitic rosary, or secondary hyperparathyroidism. Urinary phosphate excretion is large, even despite low serum phosphate values. Both a reduction in the amount of phosphate reabsorbed by the kidney and a reduction in the blood value of $1,25(OH)_2D$ are found in this disorder, and these may contribute to hypomineralization and rickets. The most successful therapeutic strategies have employed the combination of round the clock oral phosphate supplements in five divided doses provided every four hours, along with 0.25 to 0.75 μg of $1,25(OH)_2D$ every 12 hours. Oral phosphate is taken during waking hours and can be associated with diarrhea. Corrective osteotomies should be deferred until biochemical evidence of the correction of rickets is apparent. Finally, it should be noted that this condition is not a cause of hypocalcemia, but that hypophosphatemia is responsible for the rickets. These patients therefore need a treatment program which will attempt to maintain normophosphatemia for as much of the day as feasible.

Hypoparathyroidism

Hypocalcemic tetany presenting without rickets can occur in transient or permanent hypoparathyroidism. A *delayed neonatal tetany* occurs in infants who have received a cow milk based formula for several days to several weeks and is based on relative hypoparathyroidism plus the high phosphate load (and low calcium/phosphate ratio) in the formula. Human milk contains approximately 150 mg of phosphorus per liter; cow milk can have up to 1000 mg per liter. Both prepared soy and modified cow milk based formula contain 500 mg phosphorous per liter. Two factors in the infant contribute to phosphorus retention. First, the glomerular filtration rate is low in all neonates, being less than 30 ml/min/1.73 m^2. Second, PTH secretion is reduced. Thus, the high dietary load of phosphate will not be excreted efficiently and PTH-induced hypocalcemia will result. Therapy consists acutely of intravenous calcium gluconate at 200 mg/kg/dose and chronically of oral calcium lactate in the feeds to achieve a 4-to-1 calcium-to-phosphate ratio.

Idiopathic hypoparathyroidism can occur in the neonatal period or at any age in childhood. Patients manifest all the signs and symptoms of hypocalcemia mentioned earlier. Hypoparathyroidism also may occur as part of a more complex clinical picture with autoimmune endocrine failure involving the adrenals, thyroid gland, pancreas, and gastric mucosa. This syndrome also can occur in conjunction with variable T cell defects and with chronic mucocutaneous Candidiasis. This latter disorder is sometimes called the *Candida endocrinopathy syndrome*.

Hypoparathyroidism also can appear in families where it is inherited in an *autosomal dominant fashion*. The degree of hypocalcemia appears to be milder in these families.

Because the parathyroid glands arise from the III and IV pharyngeal pouches, underdeveloped parathyroids may present with abnormalities of other structures whose embryologic origin arises there: the aortic arch and the thymus. This disorder is called the *DiGeorge syndrome*, which consists of tetany, hyperphosphatemia, coarctation of the aorta, and an enormous range of T cell deficits. The major problem in these children is their aortic arch disease, and the DiGeorge syndrome should be suspected in all children with aortic arch disease and hypocalcemia, since their thymic function needs to be assessed before routine blood transfusions or live virus vaccines are used. *Surgical hypoparathyroidism* is uncommon in childhood.

The pathogenesis of hypocalcemia in hypoparathyroidism relates to a reduction in PTH secretion which both prevents the complete conversion of 25(OH)D to 1,25(OH)$_2$D and makes impossible the phosphaturic action of PTH and PTH-induced bone resorption. Thus, on balance, patients have hypocalcemia and hyperphosphatemia with hypophosphaturia. The diagnosis can be made by measurement of calcium, phosphorus, and immunoreactive PTH in serum. In addition, urinary calcium excretion is elevated (calcium/creatinine ratio greater than 0.2 mg/dl/mg/dl), phosphate excretion is diminished (% tubular reabsorption of phosphate greater than 88%) and cyclic adenosine monophosphate (cAMP) is low. Therapy with a low phosphate diet and oral 1,25(OH)$_2$D at 0.25 to 0.75 µg twice daily as well as calcium carbonate supplements will reverse hypocalcemia and hyperphosphatemia. Serum calcium should be frequently evaluated to avoid hypercalcemia.

Pseudohypoparathyroidism

Described by Fuller Albright in the 1930s, this disorder represents a failure of end-organ responsiveness to PTH. Patients have all of the features of hypocalcemic tetany, including basal ganglia calcifications and hyperphosphatemia, as well as a typical phenotype in most patients. Patients have short stature, obesity, round facies, brachydactyly, and metacarpal or metatarsal hypoplasia resulting in shortened forth and fifth fingers and toes, as well as subcutaneous calcifications. This disorder, called Albright hereditary osteodystrophy, is inherited in X-linked fashion. Other subjects have normal features but may present with osteitis fibrosa cystica. These patients have a renal nonresponsiveness to PTH, but a bone responsiveness leading to hyperparathyroid bone disease. The diagnosis is made by the presence of elevated PTH concentrations (usually two to three times normal) despite hypocalcemia. Another diagnostic test is that following PTH infusion, urinary cAMP excretion is not increased. Treatment is the same as for hypoparathyroidism.

Renal Osteodystrophy

Due to a fall in 1,25(OH)$_2$D synthesis as nephron mass is reduced, patients with renal failure develop hypocalcemia, hyperphosphatemia, increased alkaline phosphatase values and a complex form of bone disease known as renal osteodystrophy. This condition is characterized by osteitis fibrosis due to secondary hyperparathyroidism and osteomalacia due to bone undermineralization. Children demonstrate bowing and a myopathy as well as bone pain. The best form of therapy is active vitamin D metabolites to correct hypocalcemia and to suppress secondary hyperparathyroidism, calcium carbonate with meals to block intestinal phosphate absorption, and a low phosphate diet. Patients with renal osteodystrophy and chronic renal failure may have growth failure and thus any hypocalcemic child should have a blood urea nitrogen (BUN) and serum creatinine obtained in addition to the laboratory studies outlined above.

Calcium Deficiency

Rickets and hypocalcemia secondary to calcium deficiency is extremely uncommon. A calcium-deficient diet will occur as a form of child abuse, wherein the child is fed a bizarre diet, such as peanuts and Coca Cola, devoid of this mineral. An unusual form of calcium deficient osteomalacia has been described in South Africa among rural black children whose daily calcium intake is so low that they develop bone disease. Serum $1,25(OH)_2D$ values are high in these children, as are PTH levels. The addition of calcium to the diet is curative.

Magnesium Deficiency

Magnesium deficiency due to renal wasting or intestinal malabsorption can result in hypocalcemia and tetany. Autosomal recessive hypomagnesemia occurs due to an intestinal malabsorption syndrome. Some patients may have a renal leak syndrome, either with or without other tubular defects. Hypocalcemia is probably due to the impaired role of magnesium in PTH secretion and PTH-related bone resorption; thus, in the hypomagnesemic state, both PTH levels and PTH action is diminished.

Some drugs. such as cis-platin, aminoglycosides, and loop diuretics can diminish urinary magnesium reabsorption and result in hypomagnesemia. Bartter syndrome also is associated with hypermagnesuria.

The diagnosis is made by determination of serum magnesium. If reduced, urinary magnesium should be evaluated as well as PTH values. Replacement several times daily with oral magnesium oxide will reverse hypoparathyroidism hypocalcemia and tetany.

HYPERCALCEMIC DISORDERS

Hypercalcemia is far less common in childhood than in adults, particularly since the humoral hypercalcemia of malignancy is very rare in children. The symptoms of hypercalcemia very much depend on the degree of hypercalcemia with most patients with levels below 11.5 to 12 mg/dl being asymptomatic. The symptoms are lethargy, weakness, inability to concentrate mentally, and depression. Many patients have nausea, vomiting, anorexia, constipation, and weight loss. Because a high extracellular calcium concentration impairs the capacity of the distal tubule to respond to antidiuretic hormone, hypercalcemic patients have polyuria and an inability to concentrate the urine. If serum calcium rises to more than 16 mg/dl, stupor and coma may develop.

The major signs of hypercalcemia are dehydration, band keratopathy of the medial and lateral margins of the cornea, shortening of the QT interval on an electrocardiogram (EKG) recording, hypercalcuria and nephrolithiasis, pancreatitis, peptic ulcer disease and azotemia. Azotemia is related to polyuria, dehydration, nephrocalcinosis and renal stones.

In contrast to adults where malignancy and primary hyper-parathyroidism cause more than 90% of chronic hypercalcemia, a group of uncommon conditions prevail which will be discussed below.

Primary Hyperparathyroidism

Because this is a disease of adults, children rarely have sporadic primary hyperparathyroidism. This disorder is usually diagnosed by obtaining a calcium value in the elevated range or by the finding of hypercalcemia and nephrocalcinosis. Reports of bone pain, osteitis fibrosa, peptic ulcer, and hypertension are very rare in children. Due to the effect of PTH on the synthesis of $1,25(OH)_2D$, children with parathyroid adenomas have elevated serum $1,25(OH)_2D$ values, hyper-absorption of calcium from the intestine and, usually, hypercalcuria. Because a parathyroid adenoma will not regress, treatment consists of surgical extirpation of the adenoma.

Children who are members of families with the multiple endocrine neoplasia syndromes (MEN I, MEN II) should have frequent measurements of serum calcium to determine when the parathyroid adenomas are expressed. These syndromes are discussed elsewhere in Chapters 4 and 8. Most experts feel that these patients should undergo a parathyroidectomy.

While awaiting a parathyroidectomy, some children will require acute therapy of hypercalcemia. These patients should be well hydrated and furosemide will increase urinary calcium excretion. Other medications include intravenous sodium chloride, sodium sulfate, and sodium phosphate. Oral phosphate will bind calcium in the intestine, and since phosphate leads to diarrhea, of these the safest is NaCl infusions with furosemide at 1 to 2 mg/kg/dose.

Hypercalcemia of Malignancy

The usual tumors which lead to bone erosion or to humeral hypercalcemia are not found in children. Some children with leukemia may present with hypercalcemia and bony erosions. These children are usually leukopenic and have a worse prognosis than nonhypercalcemic leukemic children. In addition to the measures indicated to reduce serum calcium values, they should receive antileukemic therapy.

Children with Burkitt lymphoma also have hypercalcemia in relation to the release of certain lymphokines which increase osteoclastic bone erosion and release of mineral from bone. These lymphokines include osteoclast activating factors, interleukin 1, and others that require the action of certain prostaglandins to lead to hypercalcemia. The treatment of the underlying malignancy usually reverses hypercalcemia.

Other Endocrine Disorders Causing Hypercalcemia

Hyperthyroidism leads to active bone turnover and enhanced resorption. Hypercalcemia is mild, usually under 11 mg/dl, and disappears with appropriate therapy.

Adrenal insufficiency leads to hypercalcemia. possibly in relation to increased intestinal calcium absorption. Therapy with glucocorticoids will reverse hypercalcemia.

Familial hypocalcuric hypercalcemia is an infrequent autosomal dominant disorder that usually results in surprisingly benign symptoms despite serum calcium values as high as 15.0 mg/dl. These patients, as the name implies, have a urine calcium inappropriately low for the level of hypercalcemia. Urine calcium is under 4mg/kg/day and the calcium/creatinine ratio is usually less than 0.10. Nephrolithiasis, ulcer disease, and band keratopathy are rare. Pancreatitis can be seen in older children. A subtotal parathyroidectomy will not correct hypercalcemia.

The neonates in some kindreds may present with extremely high levels of calcium and in extremis. Serum calcium values exceeding 18.0 mg/dl are not uncommon, along with massive parathyroid hyperplasia and bone erosions. Serum $1,25(OH)_2D$ values are normal, but these children require emergency parathyroidectomy as a lifesaving procedure. This profound hypercalcemia may be present in more than one child in a sibship.

This disorder also has parathyroid hyperplasia as a common finding in all affected family members, but not to the same extent as in infants with profound hypercalcemia. For mildly affected subjects, either no therapy, a high phosphate diet, or oral phosphate supplements may be indicated.

Drug-Induced Hypercalcemia

Thiazide diuretics frequently are found to induce mild hypercalcemia, as they are natriuretic but not calciuretic. They lead to diminished urinary calcium excretion which disappears within two to three weeks after discontinuation of the drug.

Hypervitaminosis D is a condition found in children whose caregivers are health food store frequenters. Overdosage of vitamin D used to treat any of the hypocalcemic disorders will cause this finding. Hypercalcemia is particularly vexing in patients treated with ergocalciferol (vitamin D2) or cholecalciferol (vitamin D3), as these compounds are stored in fat and are released slowly into the circulation over weeks to months. Using short acting vitamin D metabolites such as 25(OH)D, 1,25(OH)$_2$D, or Hytakerol, the length of hypercalcemia is attenuated. Some patients with hypervitaminosis D may require glucocorticoids (prednisone at 1 to 2 mg/kg/day) to reduce intestinal calcium absorption.

Hypervitaminosis A also is seen in food faddists and causes hypercalcemia in relation to enhanced bone resorption. However, hypervitaminosis A rarely is found apart from hypervitaminosis D, as many preparations contain both vitamins A and D together.

The *milk alkali syndrome* consists of hypercalcemia in conjunction with the ingestion of calcium carbonate, lactate, or bicarbonate to treat peptic ulcer disease. During the past 20 years, this condition has largely disappeared, as aluminum or magnesium hydroxide-containing antacids are now used. However, in children with chronic renal insufficiency, the use of aluminum-containing phosphate-binding agents results in aluminum intoxication. Hence, physicians are turning to calcium carbonate to block intestinal phosphate accumulation. Many of these uremic children develop a new form of the milk alkali syndrome, which includes hypercalcemia, hypocalcuria, alkalosis, and all the clinical signs and symptoms of hypercalcemia.

Granulomatous Disease

Sarcoidosis is the major granulomatous disorder of childhood which results in hypercalcemia. Present evidence suggests that the sarcoid granulomas are capable of converting 25(OH)D to 1,25(OH)$_2$D, thereby causing hyperabsorption of dietary calcium and hypercalcemia. Sarcoid patients also become hypercalcemic on small doses of vitamin D, which does not induce hypercalcemia in normal children. Finally, patients with sarcoidosis have more hypercalcemia in summer months when circulating values of 25 (OH)D are higher. Glucocortoid treatment results in reduced intestinal calcium absorption, reduction in serum calcium values and a decline in 1,25(OH)$_2$D values. Other granulomatous conditions, such as tuberculosis or berylosis, have not caused hypercalcemia in children.

Miscellaneous Causes

Immobilization hypercalcemia results from enhanced bone resorption and diminished bone formation since the patient, usually a child with a fracture, is not weight bearing. Weight bearing promotes a more normal balance between bone formation and resorption. This disorder is common in adolescent males post femoral fracture in association with traction and other forms of immobilization. Treatment with intramuscular calcitonin (50 to 200 units) will block bone resorption. Ambulation of the subject is the ultimate treatment of this condition.

Idiopathic hypercalcemia of infancy is a rare disorder in which hypercalcemia is found associated with either a high vitamin D intake, as occurred in England at the end of World War II, or as a truly idiopathic condition. The mechanism of hypercalcemia is uncertain, but serum $1,25(OH)_2D$ values and $25(OH)D$ values are generally normal in children today, in contrast to those cases in the United Kingdom, where $25(OH)D$ values presumably were elevated. These children may require a low calcium diet, using a meat based formula, or even glucocorticoids for a time, but most children are asymptomatic. This condition tends to disappear with time and the patients become normocalcemic. The pathogenesis is obviously uncertain.

William syndrome was first described in the 1950s and 1960s and is a sporadic disorder consisting of short stature and developmental delay, supravalvar aortic stenosis, and a pathognomonic facial appearance. These children are said to have "elfin facies" which consists of a small head, protuberant ears, a cupid's bow lip with short philtrum, peg-like teeth, blue iris with whitish flecking, and frequent caries. They tend to be hyperactive, with a "cocktail party patter" personality. They also have an enormous discrepancy between their verbal and mathematics performance on testing and appear brighter than their full IQ scores. About 20% of these children have hypercalcemia, hypercalciuria, nephrocalcinosis, and even renal impairment. They resemble patients with hypervitaminosis D or sarcoidosis. A variety of defects have been identified in calcium metabolism in these patients, and the defects persist long after hypercalcemia has subsided. Among the defects identified are abnormal retention of oral or intravenous calcium. Elevated vitamin D3 values, abnormally high serum $25(OH)D$ values after a given load, elevated $1,25(OH)_2D$ values, elevated serum calcitonin values, and abnormal vitamin A levels. These findings, which could lead to hypercalcemia or to increased calcium retention, are still controversial.

In hypercalcemic infants with this condition, either a low calcium diet or the use of glucocorticoids to block intestinal calcium transport may be indicated. Children should use vitamin D containing compounds (vitamin capsules, diet supplements) with caution.

Fat necrosis is a rare hypercalcemic disorder in sick term or preterm infants who have had cold exposure or hypoxia. These infants have areas of fat necrosis and dystrophic calcification in their subcutaneous fat. The hypercalcemia can persist for several days to weeks if the patient survives, but it generally remits and does not lead to long-term consequences.

Suggested Readings

Bachrach S, Fisher J, Parks JS: An outbreak of vitamin D deficiency rickets in a susceptible population. Pediatrics 1979;64:871

Broadus AE: Mineral metabolism. In: Endocrinology and Metabolism. Felip P, Baxter JD, Broadus AE, Frohman LA (editors). New York: McGraw Hill, 1981, pp 963-1079

Chesney RW: Current clinical applications of vitamin D metabolite research. In: Clinical Orthopedics and Related Research. Urist MR (editor). Philadelphia: JB Lippincott Co., 1981, pp 285-314

Chesney RW, Haustra AJ, DeLuca HF, Horowitz S, Gilbert EF, Hing R, Borcherding W: Elevated serum 1,25(OH)2 vitamin D concentrations in the hypercalcemia of sarcoidosis: correction by glucocorticoid therapy. J Pediatr 1981;98:919

Chesney RW, Zimmerman J, Haustra AJ, DeLuca HF, Mazess RB: Vitamin D metabolite concentrations in vitamin D deficiency: Are calcitrol levels normal. Am J Dis Child 1981;135:1025

Chesney RW: Metabolic bone diseases. Pediatrics in Review 1984; 5:227.

Eil C, Liberman VA, Rosen JF, Marx SJ, Aurbach G: Cellular defect in hereditary vitamin D-dependent rickets type II: Defective nuclear uptake of 1,25 dehydroxyvitamin D in cultured skin fibroblasts. N Engl J Med 1981;304:1588

Fraser DS, Kooh SW, Kind HP, DeLuca HF: Pathogenesis of hereditary vitamin D dependency rickets: An inborn error of vitamin D metabolism involving defective conversion of 25-hydroxyvitamin D to 1 ,25-dehydroxyvitamin D. N Engl J Med 1978;289:817

Gloneux FM, Marie PJ, Pettifor JM et al: Bone response to phosphate salts, ergocalciferol and calcitrol in hypophosphatemia vitamin D resistant rickets. N Engl J Med 1980;303:1023

Greer FR, Chesney RW: Disorders of calcium metabolism in the neonate. Seminars in Nephrology, June 1983, pp 110-115.

Harrison HE, Harrison HC: Disorders of Calcium and Phosphate

Metabolism in Childhood and Adolescence. Philadelphia: WB Saunders, 1979, pp 53-84

Mehls O: Renal osteodystrophy in children: etiology and clinical aspects. In: End Stage Renal Disease in Children. Philadelphia: WB Saunders, 1984, pp 227-250

Marie PJ, Pettifor JM, Ross FR et al: Histologic osteomalacia due to dietary calcium deficiency in children N Engl J Med 1982;307:584

Nolten W, Chesney RW, Dabbagh S, Lemann J, Statopolsky E, Klingensmith GJ, DeLuca HF: Hypocalcemia is moderate in an asymptomatic kindred with familial hypoparathyroidism since serum 1,25(OH)2 vitamin D levels are normal. Am J Med 1987;82:1157

Rosen JF, Fleischman AR, Finberg L et al: 1,25 Dehydroxycholecalciferol: Its use in the long-term management of idiopathic hypoparathyroidism in children. J Clin Endocrinol Metab 1977;45:457

Rosen JF, Chesney RW: Circulating calcitrol concentrations in health and disease of infancy and childhood. J Pediatr 1983;103:1

Rowe JC, Wood DH, Rowe DW, Raisz L: Nutritional hypophosphatemic rickets in a premature infant fed breast milk. N Engl J Med 1979;300:293

Stelchen JJ, Tsang RC, Greer FR et al: Elevated serum 1,25 dehydroxyvitamin D concentrations in rickets of very low birthweight infants. J Pediatr 1981;99:293

Zelikovic I, Dabbagh S, Friedman AL, Goelzer ML. Chesney RW: Severe renal osteodystrophy without elevated serum immunoreactive parathyroid hormone concentrations in hypomagnesemia due to renal magnesium wasting. Pediatrics 1987;79:403

APPENDIX 7

FIGURE 7-1

THE VITAMIN D ENDOCRINE SYSTEM

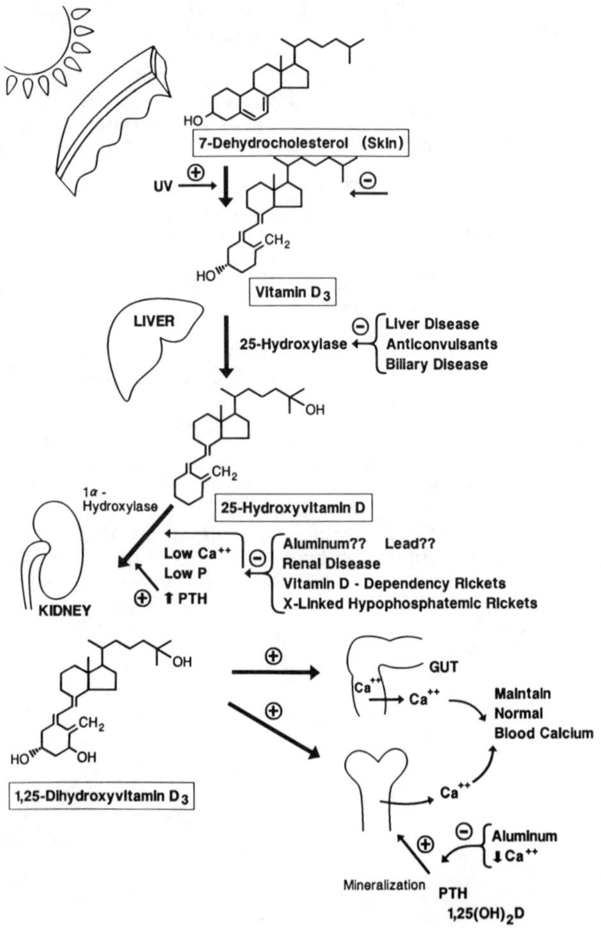

7-Dehydrocholesterol (Skin)

UV ⊕   ⊖

Vitamin D_3

LIVER

25-Hydroxylase ← ⊖ Liver Disease
Anticonvulsants
Biliary Disease

1α-Hydroxylase

25-Hydroxyvitamin D

KIDNEY

Low Ca^{++}
Low P
⊕ ↑ PTH

⊖ Aluminum??   Lead??
Renal Disease
Vitamin D - Dependency Rickets
X-Linked Hypophosphatemic Rickets

1,25-Dihydroxyvitamin D_3

⊕

⊕

Ca^{++} → Ca^{++} GUT

Maintain
Normal
Blood Calcium

Ca^{++}

⊕   ⊖ Aluminum
↓ Ca^{++}

Mineralization   PTH
1,25$(OH)_2$D

Chapter 8

Endocrine Tumors of Childhood

Endocrine tumors that fall within the purview of this chapter are those in the central nervous system (CNS) that exert influence by their mass and those in the CNS or elsewhere that secrete hormones. Hormone-secreting tumors either release hormones normally originating from the tissue encompassing the neoplasm (eutopic hormone-secreting tumors) or secrete hormones not ordinarily produced in the organ in large enough quantities to cause a biological effect (ectopic hormone secreting tumors). Some endocrine tumors of childhood are found in groups, often in a familial pattern.

CENTRAL NERVOUS SYSTEM TUMORS

Virtually any tumor of the CNS can exert pressure effects on the hypothalamic-pituitary area by enlarging or metastasizing; this can cause endocrine effects. Craniopharyngiomas are rare tumors but are the ones most commonly associated with endocrine deficiencies in the pediatric age group, compared with other types of CNS neoplasms. Other tumors in the area also can lead to pituitary deficiencies; if located in certain areas, tumors can cause increased endocrine activity, e.g., precocious puberty. Because of the range of endocrine effects of CNS tumors, they will be discussed in general in this chapter; particular endocrine effects are discussed in appropriate chapters (see Chapters 1, 2, 4, and 6).

Craniopharyngiomas are derived from Rathke's pouch and therefore arise in the pituitary stalk. They can grow upward into the hypothalamus or down into the sella turcica. Often cystic, they can contain cholesterol-laden fluid, which visually resembles motor oil. They are often calcified so that 80% show flecks of calcium on lateral skull x-ray, and more will demonstrate calcium on computerized tomographic (CT) or magnetic resonance imaging (MRI) scans of the hypothalamic-pituitary region. A child of any age may develop a craniopharyngioma, but the peak incidence is during the early teenage years. Patients will complain of headache and poor vision, they may have the polyuria and polydipsia of diabetes insipidus, their growth charts will demonstrate decreased growth velocity and, if the patient is old enough, delayed puberty may result. Physical examination will likely reveal short stature, chubbiness of hypopituitarism, pale atrophic (not dysplastic) optic disks, visual field cuts on confrontation (usually bitemporal hemianopsia), and possibly physical findings of hypothyroidism (usually subtle); there will likely be a prepubertal appearance or a cessation of the progression of secondary sexual development even in an adolescent aged patient. These historic features and signs and symptoms describe a classic patient; some have been serendipitously diagnosed by the finding of calcium flecks in the sellar area on a lateral skull x-ray taken for head trauma or orthodontia.

Germinomas of the hypothalamus are rare tumors as well but have a peak incidence in the early teenage years. The location makes any hypothalamic-pituitary deficiency possible. They may be asymptomatic except for endocrine effects such as diabetes insipidus, growth failure, and delayed puberty. Germinomas may secrete hCG and cause incomplete precocious puberty in affected boys. These tumors are radiosensitive.

HORMONE SECRETING TUMORS

Childhood neoplasms with endocrine activity may produce an excessive amount of steroid, peptide, or catecholamine, which normally is produced in physiologic concentrations in the same organ or may produce peptide hormones not usually secreted in the same organ. The disorders listed below are discussed in more detail in the chapters devoted to their organ system.

Tumors Secreting Excessive Amounts of a Hormone Which Normally Would be Produced in the Same Tissue in Physiologic Concentrations: *Eutopic Hormone Secreting Tumors*

Pituitary tissue rarely forms *adenomas* during childhood; but prolactinomas, *corticotropic adenomas* (previously called basophilic adenomas), and, most rarely of all, *somatatrope adenomas* (previously eosinophilic adenomas) are reported. Prolactinomas are treated with surgical removal if possible and bromocriptine suppression if not amenable to surgical extirpation. Basophilic and somatotrophic adenomas are removed by transsphenoidal microadenomectomy if possible.

Papillary or follicular cell carcinomas of the thyroid are nonfunctional and present on thyroid scan as cold nodules; *adenomas of the thyroid* are functional. *Medullary carcinoma of the thyroid gland* secretes calcitonin and may be a component of the multiple endocrine neoplasia syndromes.

Parathyroid adenomas may be multiple so that all parathyroid glands must be explored in affected patients. There are no malignant tumors of the parathyroid gland reported. *Hyperplasia of the parathyroid glands* can mimic the clinical presentation of parathyroid adenomas.

Islet cell adenomas of the pancreas secrete insulin and can present with symptomatic hypoglycemia; carcinoma of the pancreas may not secrete sufficient insulin to cause hypoglycemic symptoms but may secrete ectopic hormones. Islet cell tumors of the pancreas can secrete gastrin and cause the Zollinger-Ellison syndrome and gastrinomas and somatostatinomas are reported.

Adrenal adenomas or *carcinomas* can secrete excess cortisol and produce Cushing syndrome. Carcinomas can produce more virilization than adenomas. Adrenal medullary tissue can give rise to pheochromocytomas that produce a preponderance of epinephrine rather than norepinephrine.

Ovarian thecoma and *luteomas* and *arrhenoblastomas* produce virilization; *granulosa cell tumors* secrete estrogen and produce feminization. *Ovarian and adrenal androgen-secreting tumors* may present with similar clinical and laboratory features and can be identified from one another by imaging techniques or by selective vein catheterizations.

Testicular *Leydig cell tumors* secrete testosterone and cause virilization. Congenital adrenal rests in the testes may also hypertrophy under ACTH stimulation in untreated congenital adrenal hyperplasia. Testicular tumors usually can be differentiated from adrenal tumors by palpable enlargement of the testes.

Tumors Secreting Hormones not Normally Produced in Physiologic Concentrations from the Organ: Ectopic Hormone Secreting Tumors

There is evidence that protein hormones such as human chorionic gonadotropin (hCG) are produced in all tissues. This suggests that the term ectopic hormone secretion may not be appropriate for a tumor of the liver that secretes hCG; because of convention, for the purposes of this discussion, we will retain the term.

Hypothalamic germinomas or germinomas and *teratomas* of other locations can secrete hCG, which in boys will stimulate Leydig cell testosterone production. *Hepatoblastomas* and *hepatomas* also can stimulate Leydig cell function via hCG secretion. The hCG will cause the testes to be enlarged from the size found in the prepubertal state, but they will not grow as large as seen in late puberty.

Ectopic ACTH can be produced from thymomas, lung tumors, Wilm tumors and islet cell pancreatic tumors. Cushing syndrome will result from intense stimulation of the adrenal cortex and mineralocorticoid excess may cause hypokalemic alkalosis.

Pheochromocytomas may arise from chromaffin tissue in sympathetic ganglia and the organ of Zuckerkandl as well as from the adrenal medulla; extraadrenal pheochromocytomas will usually produce more norepinephrine than adrenal pheochromocytomas. Neuroblastoma and ganglioneuroma can also develop from sympathetic ganglia.

Multiple Endocrine Neoplasia Syndrome

Multiple endocrine neoplasia syndrome type 1 (*Werner syndrome*) includes hyperparathyroidism, pituitary adenomas, and pancreatic islet cell tumors. Usually pheochromocytomas are not included, but families are reported with pheochromocytoma and islet cell pancreatic tumors.

Multiple endocrine neoplasia syndrome type 2 (*Sipple syndrome*, previously called 2A) includes pheochromocytoma, medullary carcinoma of the thyroid, and hyperparathyroidism. The medullary carcinoma of the thyroid often occurs earlier and metastasizes at a younger age than occurs in sporadic medullary carcinoma of the thyroid. The pheochromocytomas are usually adrenal and may be bilateral or multicentric.

Multiple endocrine neoplasia syndrome type 3 (previously called 2B) includes pheochromocytoma, medullary carcinoma of the thyroid, and multiple mucosal neuromas, and the patient often has a Marfan syndrome-like habitus. The phenotype is quite distinctive; neuromas of the lips and tongue are most common. The physical findings should cause the physician to search for occult pheochromocytomas and medullary carcinomas of the thyroid.

Neurofibromatosis is a dominantly inherited disease of cutaneous freckles, cafe-au-lait spots, and neurofibromas. The neurofibromas may degenerate into gliomas. Hypothalamic-pituitary disorders, including growth hormone deficiency, hypogonadotropic hypogonadism, and precocious puberty are associated with tumors of the CNS. Pheochromocytomas are found in the syndrome.

Von Hippel-Lindau disease (retinal cerebellar hemangioblastomatosis) is associated with pheochromocytoma formation.

Suggested Readings

Glushien AS, Mansuy MM, Littman DS: Pheochromocytoma: Its relationship to the neurocutaneous syndromes. Am J Med 1953;14:318

Jennings MT, Gelman R, Hochberg F: Intracranial germ-cell tumors: natural history and pathogenesis. J Neurosurg 1985;63:155

Sklar CA et al: Hormonal and metabolic abnormalities associated with central nervous system germinoma in children and adolescents and the effect of therapy: report of 10 patients. J Clin Endocrinol Metab 1981;52:9

Styne DM et al: Endocrinologic, histologic, and biochemical characterization of ACTH and calcitonin producing islet cell carcinoma of the pancreas in childhood. J Clin Endocrinol Metab 1983;57:723

Thomsett MJ et al: Endocrine and neurologic outcome in childhood craniopharyngioma: review of effect of treatment in 42 patients. J Pediatr 1980;97:728

Voorhess ML: Disorders of the adrenal Medulla, multiple endocrine adenomatosis syndromes. In: Clinical Pediatric and Adolescent Endocrinology. Kaplan SA (editor). Philadelphia: WB Saunders, 1982, p 199

Woods WG, Tuchman M: Neuroblastoma: The case for screening infants in North America. Pediatrics 1987:79; 869

Chapter 9

Diabetes Mellitus

The principal form of *diabetes mellitus* that occurs in childhood and adolescence results from a deficiency of insulin secretion and is designated *insulin-dependent diabetes mellitus (IDDM)*, or *type I diabetes mellitus*, formerly referred to as juvenile-onset diabetes mellitus. A different disease results from resistance to insulin, which is designated *non-insulin-dependent diabetes mellitus (NIDDM), type II diabetes mellitus*, or *adult-onset diabetes mellitus*. NIDDM accounts for over 90% of the total cases. A comparison between these two different diseases is seen in Table 9-1.

There are acquired forms of IDDM in children resulting from pancreatic degeneration, such as cystic fibrosis. NIDDM can be found in some children with lipodystropic syndromes, ataxia telangiectasia, myotonic dystrophy, leprechaunism, Mendenhall syndrome, and acanthosis nigricans. NIDDM occurring predominantly in obese black adolescent females is referred to as maturity-onset diabetes of youth (MODY).

PATHOGENESIS

IDDM and NIDDM are genetically and clinically distinct diseases. Concordance rates for NIDDM in monozygote twins are 100% and only 20 to 50% for IDDM. It has been found that over 90% of IDDM patients have either the human lymphocyte antigen (HLA) DR_3 or DR_4 allele, or both. On the other hand, about half of the U.S. population has DR_3 or DR_4 with less than 1% developing IDDM. It is not clear how these HLA complexes produce susceptibility to diabetes. Environmental triggers are thought to convert susceptibility into disease, which is supported by the less than 50% concordance rates in identical twin studies. Viral infections, emotional stressors, and toxins all have been implicated in the expression of diabetes.

(Fig. 1). It is currently held that IDDM results from a chronic progressive autoimmune process in these susceptible individuals. The ß-cell destruction occurs over a period of months to years before the disease becomes clinically manifest. Individuals with IDDM have an increased frequency of other autoimmune diseases, such as thyroiditis, Addison disease, and rheumatoid arthritis. Although islet cell antibodies are usually present at the time of diagnosis, they have been detected in siblings during the prediabetic phase of the disease. It is still unclear whether these hallmarks of autoimmunity caused the ß-cell damage or gathered as a result of the destruction.

DIABETIC KETOACIDOSIS

Diagnosis

The clinical presentation of *diabetic ketoacidosis* usually follows a period of polyuria, polydipsia, polyphagia, and weight loss. The classic symptoms of polyuria, polydipsia, and weight loss are commonly seen along with glycosuria and ketonuria. The symptoms may have been initially associated with a viral illness that lasted longer than expected. Varying degrees of dehydration are present. There may also be abdominal pain and vomiting with diabetic ketoacidosis. With marked ketoacidosis there is deep breathing (*Kussmaul*) and a fruity odor to the breath which results from ketones. Rarely nowadays does ketosis progress to shock and coma. This combination of hyperglycemia, ketonuria, and classical symptoms are needed for the diagnosis. Glucose tolerance tests, insulin concentrations, and C-peptide measurements are not usually needed. A finding of an elevated *glycosylated hemoglobin* confirms the previous glucose intolerance. The initial laboratory tests reveal an elevated blood glucose, decreased serum bicarbonate, and positive ketones. The anion gap $[Na^+ -(HCO_3^- + Cl^-)]$ is increased above normal (14 mEq/liter) and indicates metabolic acidosis. The arterial pH is usually 7.25 or less. The total white cell count may be elevated with a marked left shift. Salicylate intoxication must be excluded since it could present a similar clinical picture.

General Principles of Diabetic Ketoacidosis Management

Hospital admission is recommended for children with the onset of their diabetes unless the symptoms are mild and close evaluation and instruction can be done outside the hospital. The child with diabetic ketoacidosis represents a medical emergency and requires close supervision during the first 24 to 48 hours of metabolic correction. The assessment of hydration, glucose levels, acidosis, and mental status needs frequent monitoring. A search for the cause of the ketoacidosis includes infection, stress, as well as omission of insulin in a previously diagnosed child. Although diabetic ketoacidosis often is associated with elevated white blood cell counts, this does not mean that infection is necessarily present. The presence of fever is a better clue to infection. With moderate dehydration, presence of pneumonia may not be appreciated on physical examination, and a chest x-ray may be diagnostic. Antibiotics should be used only for specific infection.

Diabetic ketoacidosis is a hypertonic form of dehydration. The plasma osmolality increases by 10 mOsm for every 180 mg of glucose above normal, so that the osmolality of the serum may be 320 to 350 mOsm. [Estimation of serum osmolality (mOsm/liter) = 2x serum sodium (mEq/liter) + (blood glucose (mg%)/18)]. Rehydration with normal saline (308 mOsm) should be used initially to avoid rapid fluid shifts. A change to one-half normal saline is done with the return to near normal serum osmolality. The circulatory volume is relatively well maintained with hypertonic dehydration and, thus, the deficit fluid replacement can be done evenly over a 24 to 48 hour period if the patient is not in shock.

Continuous intravenous insulin infusion, usually referred to as *low dose insulin therapy*, actually results in plasma insulin levels that are tenfold or greater than normal. The advantage of this method of insulin administration is rapid control of the plasma insulin concentration. Changes in insulin infusion will quickly alter the blood lucose.

The *cerebral edema* accident of diabetic ketoacidosis management is rare, but its sudden onset and rapid progression require constant vigilance. The correction of metabolic abnormalities may be progressing quite satisfactorily when the child shows minor behavioral changes such as crying, blinking or restlessness. It often requires a parent to detect these minimal changes, but once present, cerebral edema should be suspected and therapy to reduce intracranial pressure should be applied at once.

Protocol for Management of Diabetic Ketoacidosis

I.   Admit to intensive care unit
II. Evaluation
    A. Record vital signs along with assessment of hydration, weight, and mental status
    B. Measure blood glucose, ketones, "osmolality," pH electrolytes; obtain CBC, UA, EKG and cultures (note: ketones may cause falsely elevated creatinine by interference in some tests)
    C. Measure glucose hourly and electrolytes every four hours
III. Specific Measures
    A. Rehydration

1. If patient is in shock, administer plasma or whole blood or plasma expander and hydrocortisone (Solu-Cortef 5 to 10 mg/kg intravenously).
2. Maintenance fluid requirements:
   a. 100 ml/kg for 0-10 kg
   b. 50 ml/kg for 11-20 kg
   c. 20 ml/kg for > 20 kg
      (e.g., a 30 kg child has maintenance requirements of 1700 ml.)
3. Fluid loss:
   Estimated on the 5-10-15% basis; orthostatic changes of tachycardia are present with 10% dehydration. An ortho-static decrease in blood pressure is present with 15% or greater dehydration (e.g., moderate dehydration in a 30 kg child -- 10% of 30 kg = 3 L. Therefore, a moderately dehydrated 30 kg child requires 3 L + 1.7 L = 4.7 L in 24 hours).
4. Choice of fluid:
   a. Normal saline (308 osmol)
   b. 1/2 Normal saline (174 osmol)

Normal saline is given initially and continued until the serum osmolality reaches about 300. Glucose should not be given initially. One-half normal saline is then administered. Plan to correct the fluid deficit evenly over 24 hours. When blood glucose has fallen to less than 200 mg/100 ml, change to one-half normal saline D5W (or equivalent). As soon as patient is able to take fluids by mouth, reduce rate of intravenous therapy so that total administration will equal maintenance and losses. Discontinue intravenous therapy when patient has successfully taken fluids orally for eight hours. Then gradually introduce a soft diet.

B. Insulin Replacement
   1. Use only regular human insulin.
      a. Initial i.v. bolus dose of 0.1 unit regular insulin/kg.
      b. Continuous infusion of 0.1 unit regular insulin/kg/hr. (Insulin infusion is "piggy backed" into i.v. fluid line). To make infusion solution, add 50 units regular insulin to a 250 ml bottle of isotonic saline. Solution has 1 unit/5ml.
         (e.g., 30 kg child: 30 x 0.1 = 3 units of insulin. Infusion of 15 ml/hr will deliver 3 units of regular insulin/hr.)
   2. There should be a linear rate of decrease in blood glucose of 75 to 120 mg/hr once a steady state has been reached after the initial decrease in glucose concentration due to hydration. When the blood glucose falls below 200 mg/100

ml, the concentration of glucose in the i.v. fluid is increased to 5%.

3. When the blood glucose value falls below 150 mg%, the insulin infusion may be discontinued, or decreased to that concentration that allows a steady blood glucose concentration. With the blood glucose concentration at 150 mg% you have the option of maintaining the i.v. insulin infusion at a lower insulin dose until the patient is able to eat or until the usual daily insulin dose would be taken.

Example: A known diabetic child is admitted to the ward at 9:00 PM and has a blood sugar of 150 mg% at 2:00 AM. Rather than switch to subcutaneous insulin, the patient is maintained on intravenous insulin at about 0.025 units/kg/hr and one-half normal saline with 5% glucose until morning, when the usual dose of regular and NPH insulin will be given before breakfast.

Example: Diabetic children having general anesthesia and surgery are more easily managed during the procedure and postoperative period, with a continuous intravenous insulin infusion and one-half normal saline with 5% glucose until ready to establish a regular eating pattern.

Example: A newly diagnosed child with diabetes has been treated for ketoacidosis, and the blood sugar is now 150 mg%. The patient is taking oral feedings and feeling well enough to start meals. Insulin should be calculated to cover feeding during the day. Start with 0.5 units of regular insulin/kg/day as the baseline and divide into four doses to be administered subcutaneously during the day. A 30 kg child would need 15 units per day divided into one-third at breakfast, one-quarter at noon, one-third at dinner and one-twelfth at bedtime.

15 units baseline insulin (0.5 units/kg)

	breakfast	lunch	dinner	bedtime
Portion	1/3	1/4	1/3	1/12
U of regular insulin	5	4	5	1

In addition, a sliding rule of regular insulin is added to or sub-tracted from each dose based on an algorithm.

Typical Algorithm for Short-term Insulin Correction
(Sliding Scale)

Blood Sugar	Instruction for use of regular insulin
less than 60 mg/dl	omit regular, recheck glucose after meal
60 - 80 mg/dl	decrease regular 10%
80 - 120 mg/dl	usual dose
120 - 180 mg/dl	increase by 10%
180 - 240 mg/dl	increase by 15%
240 - 300 mg/dl	increase by 20%
greater than 300 mg/dl	increase by 30% and check urinary ketones

This is intended only as a start and the total insulin dose of 0.5 unit/kg may require adjustment.

C. Acidosis;
   If serum bicarbonate level is less than 7, or pH is less than 7.0, it is recommended to give bicarbonate every four hours until serum bicarbonate level is 12 mmol/liter. The following formula may be used:

   (12 minus observed bicarbonate value) X 0.6 body weight (kg) = amount of sodium bicarbonate required to correct bicarbonate value to 12.

   Half of this amount may be infused in 30 minutes and the remainder over the next two hours.

D. Potassium Replacement;

One of the greatest single problems in diabetic coma is hypokalemia. In ketoacidosis there is always a deficit in total body potassium.

1. A raised serum potassium indicates a mild deficit.
2. A normal serum potassium indicates a moderate deficit.
3. A low serum potassium indicates a severe deficit.
   a. Commence replacement of potassium by adding 26 mEq (2 g)/liter i.v. fluid when:
      (1) Blood glucose is falling
      (2) Ketones are disappearing from the plasma
      (3) Adequate urinary output
   b. Monitor changes in potassium by serial biochemical determinations and electrocardiograms.
   c. Administer additional potassium as necessary to a maximum of 70-100 mEq/hour (20-80 mEq/liter) if:
      (1) Initial serum potassium is low
      (2) Electrocardiographic or biochemical evidence of hypokalemia
   d. Aim to keep the serum potassium greater than 3mEq/liter. Remember that:
      (1) Expansion of extracellular volume
      (2) Correction of acidosis or development of alkalosis
      (3) Administration of saline
      (4) Falling blood glucose levels
      (5) Glucose and insulin administration
      (6) Exchange of intracellular sodium for extracellular potassium.

All favor the development of hypokalemia; therefore, treat vigorously but *note*: Too much potassium given too fast may be lethal. The usual helpful physical signs, e.g., peripheral reflexes or bowel mobility may be deceptive as a guidelines and should not be relied upon. Also, take care if there is evidence of compromised renal function.

IV. Progress
   A. Continue daily measurements of serum electrolytes
   B. Examine urine for infection and treat energetically
   C. When the blood glucose levels are stabile, take 2/3 of the total of the morning and lunchtime insulin requirement. Administer this amount as a single dose of intermediate acting insulin before breakfast. Do the same with dinner and evening dose and administer before dinner.

D. Initial improvement followed by deterioration is usually due to:
1. uncorrected acidosis
2. hypokalemia
3. hypoglycemia
4. persistent hypotension or gram negative infections
5. cerebral edema

This must be sought for and treated. The patient who shows biochemical normalization, yet whose mental state deteriorates, may have cerebral edema.

Treat by
1. hyperventilation
2. mannitol infusion
3. glucocorticoids

OUTPATIENT MANAGEMENT OF THE CHILD WITH DIABETES

During the initial hospitalization, the family is not ready for intensive education in diabetes. Family members need time to get over the shock, relief, and grief associated with the diagnosis. Therefore, only survival skills are given at this time. Blood glucose monitoring before each meal and bedtime, urine ketone testing each morning, and record keeping should be mastered along with insulin preparation and administration. This, along with recognition and treatment of hypoglycemic symptoms should be taught to both parents. The emphasis on blood glucose monitoring before meals is to determine the next insulin dose. This gives the family a reason for its use. Tight control of blood glucose should not be a goal during the hospital stay as the home setting will be quite different. The use of only regular insulin for a couple of hospital days allows the patient and both parents more opportunity to demonstrate their skill. Once proficient in these steps, the child is discharged, and daily telephone contact is carried out for a couple of weeks. Many questions and concerns arise during this time, and it is now that all are more receptive to an education program.

The ambulatory education program is best managed using a team approach. The physician, the nurse educator, the dietician, and the patient are the team. The child's nutritional requirements are similar to other children of the same age. The calorie composition of 50% carbohydrate, 30% fat, and 20% protein is incorporated into a meal plan. This meal plan is translated into exchanges according to the American Diabetes Association. Although three meals and three snacks are recommended, individual modification of the diet is done by the dietician. The important principle for successful insulin therapy is constancy in the timing and amount of calorie intake and activity.

The most frequently used insulin regimen is the twice-daily injection of combined short-acting and intermediate-acting insulin (Fig. 3). Approximately two-thirds of the total daily insulin is given before breakfast for day time coverage. About one-half to two-thirds of this dose is the short-acting insulin. When short acting-insulin is administered subcutaneously the serum peak is reached in about two hours. Ideally, this insulin would be given 30 minutes before the meal. The intermediate-acting insulins have a peak activity around eight hours following injection. Examples of short-acting insulin are regular or semilente insulin. Intermediate-insulins include NPH and lente. The new purified or single peak insulins are preferred in children because of the lessened antigenicity and long term need. Normalization of the lunch or bedtime blood glucose level may require change in the short-acting insulin. (Fig. 3a) Normalization of the breakfast and dinner glucose level may require change in the intermediate-acting insulins. Evening intermediate-acting insulin adjustments should be made only after a two to four A.M. blood glucose value has been obtained. It should be increased only if this value is greater than 70 mg%. Inability to normalize the morning blood sugar may require a delay in administration of the intermediate-acting insulin to bedtime (Fig. 3b).

Another insulin regimen uses a long-acting or ultra-insulin along with regular insulin before each meal (Fig. 3c). The ultra-insulin dose is approximately 50% of the total daily insulin need. This is then divided and given with the short-acting insulin dose before breakfast and before dinner. A third dose of short-acting insulin is administered before lunch. The ultrainsulin does not have a defined peak but has the disadvantage of prolonged activity beyond 24 hours. This may build up resulting in unexplained hypoglycemia.

A remission or *honeymoon* phase of diabetes is present in some children after the onset. The total daily insulin dose decreases to less than 0.5 U/kg and indicates the return of some endogenous insulin secretion. This may continue for weeks to months, but endogenous insulin secretion is usually absent by the end of the first year. Endogenous insulin secretion can be monitored by the measurement of urinary C-peptide excretion, because administered insulin does not contain a C-peptide fragment. The daily insulin requirement is 0.5 to 1 U/kg with the loss of endogenous insulin secretion. During adolescence this daily dose may be 1.5 U/kg or greater.

Good metabolic control of diabetes cannot be achieved without attention to psychosocial factors. Despite the level of knowledge, the family and patient must be seen and supported at three to four month intervals. The permanency of the diabetes with no vacations or weekends off, the frustration of not understanding wide swings in blood glucose levels, and the fear of hypoglycemia are present in all. The adolescent confronts the restrictions imposed by diabetes in all phases of achieving independence. Dealing with the psychosocial issues is an important responsibility of team management.

SHORT-TERM COMPLICATIONS

Ambulatory education includes *sick day* insulin management to correct diabetic ketoacidosis. Despite nausea and vomiting, insulin is needed. The stress of the illness stimulates insulin counter-regulatory hormones that usually increase the insulin requirement. It is recommended that the intermediate-acting insulin be omitted and only the short-acting insulin be given at two to four hour intervals to decrease the blood glucose and decrease the urine ketones on these days. With correction of the blood glucose, the vomiting and nausea will stop and the usual insulin dose resumed. The patient and family are taught algorithms for insulin adjustments based on blood glucose and anticipated activities (as noted above).

Recognition of the *Somogyi* phenomenon is important in children. Nocturnal hypoglycemia followed by rebound hyperglycemia may produce night terrors, night sweats, and morning headaches. The elevated morning glucose should not be treated with an increase in the evening intermediate-acting insulin dose until an insulin-waning effect has been established with a 2:00 to 4:00 AM blood glucose value. Exercise hypoglycemia may be avoided over the short term by taking one carbohydrate exchange every 30 minutes. The subcutaneous injection of glucagon is used for hypoglycemia when the patient is uncooperative or unconscious.

LONG-TERM ASSESSMENT

Growth and development are assessed at every visit. The glycosylated hemoglobin level should be obtained at two to three month intervals to look at long-term control. Yearly measurements of thyroid function, cholesterol, triglycerides, and renal function are done. Regular dental care and ophthalmologic examinations are encouraged. Exercise programs, diabetic camps, and local diabetic groups are supportive and informative for the maintenance of good metabolic control.

Suggested Reading

Amiel AS, Tamborlane WV: New treatment methods in diabetes mellitus. in Current Concepts in Pediatric Endocrinology. Styne DM, Brook CGD (editors). Elsevier New York: 1987, p126

Eisenbarth GS: Type I diabetes mellitus: A chronic autoimmune disease. N Engl J Med 1986;314:1360

Foster D, McGarry D: The metabolic derangements and treatment of diabetic ketoacidosis. N Eng J Med 1983;309:159

Rotter JI, et. al: HLA genotype study of insulin dependent diabetes: The excess of DR3/DR4 heterozygotes allows rejection of the recessive hypothesis. Diabetes 1983;32:169

Sperling MA: Diabetes Mellitus. in Clinical Pediatric and Adolescent Endocrinology. Kaplan SA (editor) Philadelphia: WB Saunders 1982, p-131

Travis LB, Brouhard BH, Schreiner B Diabetes Mellitus in Children and Adolescents Philadelphia: WB Saunders, 1987

APPENDIX 9

TABLE 9-1

CHARACTERISTICS OF DIABETES

CLINICAL	IDDM	NIDDM
Appearance of onset	lean	obese
Peak age at onset	12-14 years	>50 years
Clinical presentation	polyuria, polydipsia and weight loss over 2-4 weeks	insidious
Ketosis	usual	uncommon
Incidence	0.1-0.3/1000/yr	accounts for >90% of diabetes
Pathogenesis	pancreatic islet cell changes leading to eventual loss of insulin	pancreatic insulin secretion but development of insulin resistance
Genetics	HLA types DR_3 & DR_4	
Islet cell antibody	positive	negative

APPENDIX 9

FIGURE 9-1

PATHOGENESIS OF IDDM

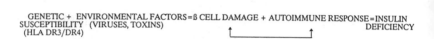

GENETIC + ENVIRONMENTAL FACTORS = ß CELL DAMAGE + AUTOIMMUNE RESPONSE = INSULIN
SUSCEPTIBILITY   (VIRUSES, TOXINS)   DEFICIENCY
(HLA DR3/DR4)

FIGURE 9-2

CLINICAL PHASES OF INSULIN DEPENDENT DIABETES

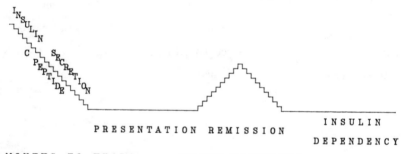

PRESENTATION   REMISSION   INSULIN
                                        DEPENDENCY

MONTHS TO YEARS   WEEKS TO MONTHS

FIGURE 9-3

INSULIN TREATMENT REGIMENS

<u>SHORT</u>   <u>SHORT</u>
  <u>INTERMEDIATE</u>   <u>INTERMEDIATE</u>

a. B   L   D   BT   B
    ^   ^

<u>SHORT</u>   <u>SHORT</u>
  <u>INTERMEDIATE</u>   <u>INTERMEDIATE</u>

b. B   L   D   BT   B
    ^   ^   ^

<u>SHORT</u>   <u>SHORT</u>   <u>SHORT</u>
  <u>LONG</u>

c. B   L   D   BT   B
    ^   ^   ^

^ = Insulin injection times

SHORT = Regular or semilente insulin action
INTERMEDIATE = NPH or lente insulin action
LONG = Ultralente insulin action

B = breakfast
L = lunch
D = dinner
BT= bedtime

Chapter 10

Hypoglycemia

Hypoglycemia may be precipitated from various endocrine disorders, from other abnormalities of metabolism, from excessive endogenous or exogenous insulin, and from vagaries of a feeding schedule. The causes of hypoglycemia vary in frequency with age, as one etiology may be of great importance in the neonate but very unlikely to occur in the teenager.

NORMAL CARBOHYDRATE METABOLISM

The maintenance of normal blood sugar depends upon (a) the *intake of carbohydrates* from the gastrointestinal tract; (b) *gluconeogenesis*, or the production of glucose from precursors such as glycerol (derived from fat), amino acids (such as alanine) and factors of anaerobic glycolysis (such as lactate and pyruvate); and (c) *glycogenolysis* or the release of glucose from its storage depot, glycogen. Glucose production and utilization is about 5 to 7 mg/kg/min in infants and young children as compared to 1 to 2 mg/kg/min in the adult; thus, an impairment in production with no change in utilization will lower glucose concentration more quickly in the child than the adult. Further, as the brain is much larger for body size in the infant than in the adult, neurologic symptoms and signs of hypoglycemia will be manifest more readily in the child. The muscle mass is smaller in children and the release of substrates of gluconeogenesis is more limited. Thus, for many reasons, the child is then more susceptible to hypoglycemia than is the adult. Conversely, if the child has brain damage resulting in lower metabolic needs for this organ that normally utilizes so much glucose, hyperglycemia may result.

After a meal, in the postprandial state, exogenous glucose is utilized by, and stored in, tissues while the mechanism of glucose production, gluconeogenesis, is decreased. Thus, insulin rises and glucagon falls with glucose intake.

The liver and kidneys are the organs that contain the enzymes necessary for *gluconeogenesis* and also the enzyme that allows the release of glucose into the circulation during *glycogenolysis*, glucose-6-phosphatase; except for states of severe starvation, the liver plays the major role in gluconeogenesis and glycogenolysis. The liver can also form the ketone bodies, acetoacetate and ß-hydroxy-butyrate. Glucose can be utilized by other tissues in various ways: anaerobic glycolysis (the Embden-Meyerhof pathway) in muscle will produce pyruvate, which is metabolized to lactate or alanine which in turn can be used as gluconeogenic precursors: oxidation of glucose to glycerol-3-phosphate in adipose tissue will esterify fatty acids to synthesize triglycerides or alternatively produce fatty acids: oxidation through acetyl-CoA in the brain will produce carbon dioxide and water. In states of low glucose availability, the energy needs of some organs can shift to conserve glucose: the liver, adipose tissue, and muscle can use the ß-oxidation of fatty acids; the brain can utilize ketone bodies.

The concentration of glucose in the serum of normal subjects is kept remarkably constant by *glucoregulatory factors*. *Insulin* is secreted from the ß cells of the pancreatic islets in response to exogenous glucose and, in turn, suppresses endogenous glucose production by inhibiting hepatic glycogenolysis and gluconeogenesis. Insulin is a potent suppressor of ketone body formation. Further, insulin stimulates storage of glucose as glycogen and triglycerides and promotes the uptake of glucose in many other tissues, such as muscle and kidney. *Glucagon* is released from the α cells of the pancreas and quickly but transiently stimulates glycogenolysis and gluconeogenesis. *Epinephrine* rapidly stimulates hepatic glycogenolysis and gluconeogenesis and acts as well through adrenergic mechanisms indirectly affecting insulin and glucagon. Both *cortisol* and *growth hormone* exert anti-insulin effects by limiting glucose utilization and increasing glucose production. Growth hormone, however, through the production the somatomedins or insulin-like growth factors, has an additional effect of lowering glucose, although the glucose elevating effect usually predominates.

HYPOGLYCEMIA

Symptoms of *hypoglycemia* are due either to effects of epinephrine secreted from the adrenal medulla (causing sweating, tremulousness, and tachycardia) or to central nervous system manifestations (such as headaches or reduced mentation, which may extend on a continuum from drowsiness to coma and seizures). If severe and recurrent hypoglycemia is ultimately controlled, the patient still may be left with permanent neurologic impairment such as mental retardation and seizure disorders that manifest even when the blood sugar is normal. Patients on adrenergic blocking agents may not show the initial symptoms of hypoglycemia in spite of having low blood sugar concentrations and they still have the potential for neurologic damage.

Hypoglycemia in the Newborn

The definition of hypoglycemia is based upon statistical analysis of the normal range of glucose values and, in the newborn especially, standards change with respect to clinical condition. Most pediatricians accept Cornblath's definition of hypoglycemia in the low birth weight infant to be values <20 mg/dl, in the full term infant during the first three days after birth to be values <30mg/dl and thereafter to be values <40 mg/dl (add 5 mg/dl to the standards if serum or plasma glucose is measured by the laboratory rather than blood glucose). Symptoms of hypoglycemia in the newborn range from grand mal or localized seizures to irritability, hypotonia, lethargy, difficulty in feeding to other rather nonspecific findings or no findings at all. Because a hypoglycemic infant may have no symptoms, routine glucose monitoring is performed in certain clinical conditions known to be associated frequently with hypoglycemia.

The neonate has less tolerance to fasting and stress than an older individual, and hypoglycemia develops faster in the newborn. Disorders causing hypoglycemia in the newborn can be found on a continuum from decreased ability to stabilize metabolically in the postnatal period, continuing to hypoglycemia as a secondary finding associated with other diseases, and ending with disorders in which severe, unremitting hypoglycemia is the immediate and primary problem. A neonate who is the product of a problem pregnancy or delivery is a likely candidate for *transient hypoglycemia*. Thus, infants who are premature or small for gestational age, or who experienced trauma, asphyxia, or cold exposure at birth should be monitored prospectively for the development of hypoglycemia. Diseases that have other significant manifestations may have hypoglycemia included in the constellation; frequent examples include sepsis, post exchange transfusion or erythroblastosis fetalis, congenital heart disease, or congenital defects of the CNS or elsewhere. The condition of the mother prior to delivery may affect the neonate as well; infants of mothers with toxemia, with narcotic addiction, taking oral hypoglycemic agents or ß-adrenergic blockers, or receiving a large amount of intravenous glucose (which will reach the fetus but will be abruptly discontinued at the time of placental separation) are likely candidates for hypoglycemia. Infants of mothers with permanent or gestational diabetes mellitus experience intrauterine hyperglycemia and develop islet cell hyperplasia due to stimulation by ambient glucose concentrations; after birth, when removed from maternal glucose, the increased insulin secretion will cause minimal to severe hypoglycemia for hours to days after delivery. The child has a characteristic appearance with extra subcutaneous tissue, a plethoric complexion, and a rather lethargic level of activity.

Newborns with *persistent hypoglycemia* who require   more than 10 to 12mg/kg/min of intravenous glucose to maintain a normal blood sugar will have more difficult problems than those mentioned above. Permanent hyperinsulinism may be caused by *islet cell adenoma*, the hyperinsulinism of the *Beckwith-Weideman syndrome* (exomphalos, macroglossia and gigantism), or *infant giants* (large body size and microcephaly but no macroglossia or exomphalos). *Neisidioblastosis* has been classically described as the development of ß-cell islets from pancreatic duct tissue but recent histologic studies suggest that this appearance is a normal variant; perhaps some of the patients previously diagnosed as having neisidioblastosis have microscopic adenomas that have been missed or a functional defect that cannot be demonstrated histologically. Deficiencies of growth hormone and/or ACTH may cause neonatal hypoglycemia and in boys the occurrence of microphallus (due to gonadotropin and growth hormone deficiency) and hypoglycemia should strongly suggest this diagnosis; visual impairment and optic hypoplasia also may be found in this constellation. Metabolic abnormalities of branched chain amino acids such as *maple syrup urine disease* (or *methylmelonic aciduria*) or carbohydrate metabolism may manifest in the newborn or older child. Screening for *galactosemia* is carried out in most neonatal screening programs, but the other possibilities, such as *glycogen storage disease type 1*, must be considered individually.

Hypoglycemia in Older Children

Many of the same conditions noted under the newborn can be diagnosed initially as causes of hypoglycemia in later life, although there will be a change in the incidence of the disorders with advancing age. Hyperinsulinism will be more likely due to a *β-cell adenoma* after the newborn period, especially after the age of three years. *Glycogen storage disease (GSD)* other than type 1 becomes more common at an older age.

Ketotic hypoglycemia classically presents in a thin (often male) child who has had a longer than average overnight fast (called the Saturday night-Sunday morning syndrome because of the purported late return of parents at night, causing a late breakfast the following morning). This term is quite general and includes many nonhyperinsulinemic causes of hypoglycemia, including growth hormone and ACTH deficiency; after reviewing the history, it may become clear that the child had neonatal hypoglycemia, which apparently resolved after regular feedings were started. Some studies have shown that affected patients tolerate an 18-hour fast more poorly than unaffected patients and that there may be an associated defect in the mobilization of alanine for gluconeogenesis.

Several types of glycogen storage diseases (GSD) cause hypoglycemia of various types. *GSD type 1* is due to a hepatic defect in glucose-6-phosphatase eliminating effective gluconeogenesis and glycogenolysis. Presentation of hypoglycemia may be in the neonatal period or later after the development of characteristic growth failure and hepatomegaly (kidneys are also large). *GSD type 3* is due to a deficiency in amylo-1,6-glucosidase, the debrancher enzyme for glycogenolysis; this is a milder condition than GSD type 1. GSD type 6 is due to phosphorylase deficiency and also leads to hypoglycemia and hepatomegaly but is also a milder condition than GSD type 1. *Hereditary fructose intolerance* is due to a defect in fructose-1-phosphate aldolase. Affected patients have severe vomiting, diarrhea, and failure to thrive when exposed to fructose, although they are normal if fructose is restricted. Children with fructose 1-6 diphosphatase deficiency have hypoglycemia when exposed to fructose, alanine, glycerol, sorbitol, and lactate as well as during infections or severe starvation.

Other causes of hypoglycemia include *malnutrition* due to gastrointestinal disease, *alcohol ingestion*, *ackee fruit ingestion* (*Jamaican vomiting disease*), *Reye syndrome* or other causes of hepatic failure and the use of drugs that have hypoglycemia as a side effect, such as aspirin or oral hypoglycemic agents; *propranolol* can cause hypoglycemia, especially after a fast, for example, when it is used to augment the response to a growth hormone provocative test after an overnight fast.

Diagnosis of Hypoglycemia

Attention should be directed toward anticipating the possibility that hypoglycemia may occur so that less effort is required toward the diagnosis and treatment of the condition. Thus, patients with stressful deliveries, with prematurity, intrauterine growth retardation, or, conversely, infants with large body size suspected to be the product of a mother with diabetes mellitus, all should have blood sugars monitored at frequent intervals during the first 24 hours after birth.

In older patients, the pattern of hypoglycemia is of extreme importance in the differential diagnosis. Fasting hypoglycemia more likely will indicate a defect in glucose production, such as a defect in gluconeogenesis or a glycogen storage disease, whereas postprandial (or reactive) hypoglycemia suggests a hyperinsulinemic state; there is overlap, however. Further, the presence of ketones in the urine or blood at the time of hypoglycemia will reflect the insulin secretory state; ketotic hypoglycemia is virtually incompatible with hyperinsulinism but nonketotic hypoglycemia increases the likelihood that insulin is not being secreted as an etiologic agent in the condition.

When a child is experiencing hypoglycemia, a blood sample should be obtained immediately so that determinations crucial to the diagnosis can be ordered. Glucose is then given to raise blood sugar; the hypoglycemic episode should not be dangerously protracted just to obtain blood for the diagnostic sample, however. The aim of management of a hypoglycemic child is to prevent the recurrence of hypoglycemia; metabolic derangements causing hypoglycemia are ideally monitored at the time of the first documented episode. If no diagnosis has been suggested by the history or physical appearance, the blood sample obtained during the hypoglycemic episode should be sent for glucose, insulin, ketone bodies, cortisol, growth hormone, lactate, pyruvate, and amino acid screen; serum should be frozen for future determinations should one area of diagnostic possibility seem more fruitful after the initial results are back.

If no diagnosis is made on the initial sample, several steps should follow. Frequent measurement of blood glucose is made during a 24-hour period, before each meal and at one, two, three hours after one or two meals and in the middle of the night. If the blood sugar is decreased, as reflected by a fingerstick glucose method, on any of these samples, the full set of tests noted above are performed before glucose is given to raise the blood sugar concentration. Of particular importance is an insulin determination, which should be determined contemporaneously with a glucose concentration. If no episode of spontaneous hypoglycemia occurs, a fast should be performed with fingerstick blood sugar monitoring.

The child should be prepared with a *high carbohydrate diet* for three days prior to the fast. The fast should start after a usual overnight period of sleep (if the child usually goes without food at night) so that the 10th to 12th hour of the routine fast starts at 7:00 to 8:00 AM, a time when the hospital staff should be around to handle complications. Fingerstick glucose determinations are made every two hours until there is a tendency for a drop in glucose. At that time, laboratory glucose determinations are made at the same time as the fingerstick samples, and urine ketones should be noted carefully to see if ketosis is developing. If the fast is demonstrating no drop in glucose by 5:00 PM (after 20 to 22 hours), the test can be continued for a full 24 hours if adequate staff is available to monitor the child safely. If the glucose concentration drops to less than 60 mg/dl, glucagon at a dose of 30μg/kg to a maximum of 1 mg is given and after 10 minutes blood glucose, insulin, lactate, and pyruvate are measured to see if there are adequate glycogen stores. The fast is usually stopped by 24 hours, and if no hypoglycemia is demonstrated, it is at least apparent that the child can tolerate a 24-hour fast at home, although such a long fast is not, of course, recommended.

Various tolerance tests are used in the differential diagnosis of hypoglycemia. The *leucine* (orally, dissolved in a slurry of CO_2-free water administered through a stomach tube, at 150 mg/kg or intravenously 75 mg/kg and blood obtained for glucose and insulin at 5, 10, 20, 30, 45, 60, 90, and 120 minutes or every 10 minutes for an hour, respectively) or the *tolbutamide tolerance test* (20-30 mg/kg up to 1 gram intravenously and blood sampled at 5, 10, 20, 30, 45, 60, 90, and 120 minutes) will determine if insulin secretion is inappropriately high but the tests may be dangerous, as severe hypoglycemia may be precipitated by the insulin secretagogues. The *glucagon tolerance test* (30 μg/kg intravenously or intramuscularly with glucose – free fatty acids, ketones, insulin, and growth hormone determinations obtained at 0, 5, 15 and 15 minutes thereafter for two hours) determines whether glycogen can be broken down to supply glucose; used in the fed or fasting state, there will be no rise in glucose in glycogen storage disease type 1 (glucose-6-phosphatase deficiency), whereas in ketotic hypoglycemia or glycogen storage disease type 3 there will be a normal response in the fed state and a poor response after a fast. The fructose tolerance test is used to evaluate hereditary fructose intolerance or 1,6-diphosphatase deficiency; because of gastrointestinal symptoms, the intravenous test is preferred: 0.25g/kg/5 min is given with a resulting fall in glucose (specific measures must be used so that reducing substances do not change the results) and inorganic phosphorus with a rise in plasma magnesium and uric acid in affected children. The *glucose tolerance test* is rarely indicated, but if performed to rule out reactive hypoglycemia, it is important to carry out several important procedures to ensure that false results do not confuse the issue: (1) three days of high carbohydrate diet must be ingested or the response to the oral glucose load will be falsely abnormal even if the patient is normal (this type of preparation is also important for the other tolerance tests listed above; (2) an insulin determination should accompany each glucose measurement; (3) the test should extend for 5 hours to look for late hypoglycemia that would be missed on a shorter test; and (4) the dose of glucose is 1.75 g/kg as a 20% solution. Symptomatology of the patient should be recorded during the test so that any low blood sugar determinations can be matched with symptoms of hypoglycemia.

The method of *measurement of glucose* also deserves attention. Methods measuring reducing substances, such as Clinitest, will measure other substances, such as galactose, whereas those using a glucose oxidase technique will be specific for glucose. Methods measuring whole blood glucose will report values that are 15% lower than those using plasma glucose. Fingerstick methods of assessing blood glucose are available, and results are read colorimetrically by comparing the color on the strip of paper containing the reagents to a color chart. The colors can be compared visually or a colorimetric machine can be used to read the value; although the machine will give an extra degree of accuracy, its use is usually unnecessary for the purposes of diagnosing or treating hypoglycemia unless the parents cannot learn how to read the color strips. The color strips must be considered supportive evidence of the glucose level as the condition and age of the strip as well as the patient's technique can change the result, generally in a lower direction. Critical values must be determined by a blood or plasma glucose reading at a licensed laboratory. The method of determining blood glucose depends upon the way in which the sample was collected. If an empty tube (red top) is used to collect the blood, metabolic activity in the sample can reduce the concentration of glucose significantly over several hours. Thus, any sample collected in an empty tube must be analyzed soon after collection. Tubes containing fluoride (grey top), which stop any glucose metabolism and allow the storage of blood for hours without lowering the glucose concentration, are preferable.

The Treatment of Hypoglycemia

The initial treatment of hypoglycemia must be glucose sufficient to bring the blood glucose to adequate levels to return neurologic function to normal. In a child who is only moderately symptomatic, *oral glucose* is adequate; table sugar, honey (if the child is over 1 year of age), or jelly can be administered to the child's buccal mucosa if the child is too disoriented to swallow. For more severe hypoglycemia, *intravenous glucose* is necessary. Dextrose in water is given in 25% concentration as a bolus of 1 ml/kg. If more dextrose in higher concentration is administered, there is a risk of hyperosmolality developing. Once the blood sugar is raised, the child should be watched; if the sugar again decreases, an infusion of dextrose, 5 to 10% should be started; there must be sodium chloride in the infusion to avoid hyponatremia developing as the hypoglycemia is repaired. It is useful to calculate the amount of glucose in terms of mg/kg/min to determine how severe the hypoglycemia is. If more than 12 to 15 mg/kg/min of glucose is required, the child has severe hypoglycemia, most likely due to hyperinsulinism.

Other measures are used for the management of severe hypoglycemia. *Diazoxide*, a benzothiodiazine hypotensive agent, in doses of 5 to 20 mg/kg/day divided into a dose every six hours will suppress insulin secretion in some cases of hyperinsulinism. Diazoxide has been used for years in the management of some conditions but will not usually be useful in ß-cell adenomas. A lack of response to diazoxide is not diagnostic but does suggest the presence of a ß-cell adenoma that will require surgical removal. *Pancreatectomies* have in the past generally limited to 80% removal, but 95% pancreatectomies are becoming more common if a definite adenoma cannot be found and removed with an 80% pancreatectomy. *Corticosteroids* also have been useful in raising blood sugar but should not be used for long term replacement except in cases of cortisol or ACTH deficiency. *Growth hormone therapy* is offered in cases of growth hormone deficiency. Of most importance in therapy is the speedy institution of a treatment designed to raise blood sugar and guard against severe and repetitive hypoglycemia and thereby to salvage mental function.

Suggested Readings

Burton BK: Inborn errors of metabolism: The clinical diagnosis in early infancy. Pediatrics 1987;79:359

Stanley CA, Baker L: Hyperinsulinism in infants and children: diagnosis and therapy. In: Adv Pediatr 1976;32:315

Cornblath M, Schwartz R: Disorders of Carbohydrrate Metabolism in Infancy. Philadelphia: WB Saunders, 1976.

Grant DB, Dunger DB, Burns EC: Long-term treatment with diazoxide in childhood hyperinsulinism. Acta Endocrinol Suppl 1986;279:340

Langer JC, et al: Surgical management of persistent neonatal hypoglycemia due to islet cell dysplasia. J Pediatr Surg 1984;19:786

LaFranchi S: Hypoglycemia of infancy and childhood. Pediatr Clin North Am 1987;34:961

Lovinger RD, Kaplan SL, Grumbach MM: Congenital hypopituitarism associated with neonatal hypoglycemis and microphallus: four cases secondary to hypothalmic hormone deficiency. J Pediatr 1975;87:1171

Pagliara AS, et al: Hypoglycemia in infancy and childhood. J Pediatr 1973;32:305, 558

Phillip M, Bashan N, Smith CP, Moses SW: An algorithmic approach to diagnosis of hypoglycemia. J Pediatr 1987;110:387

Chapter 11

Obesity

The incidence of obesity in children has increased more than 50% during the last 20 years, according to analysis of Department of Health Education and Welfare statistics. Much to the dismay of many physicians and parents, obesity is rarely the result of an endocrine disease or, in fact, any diagnosable disorder. Although there may be metabolic abnormalities in the obese patient, it will be the patient's oral intake and energy expenditure that will determine the weight of the patient, and no pill or short-term therapy will resolve the condition. It is no wonder that treatments for and books about obesity are among the top growth industries in the United States, with billions of dollars devoted to the cure, recure and multiple more cures of obesity. The wild variety of "diets" and books on the subject should attest to the lack of a unifying, effective, and lasting approach to the condition.

ADIPOSE TISSUE METABOLISM

The mass of adipose tissue is often considered an organ because of its important influence upon metabolism and its influence as a source of energy. The *adipose organ* is a reservoir of triglycerides, high-energy compounds that yield 9 kcal of energy per gram of tissue, more than twice as much energy as carbohydrate, which yields 4 kcal/g. The adipose organ accumulates more triglycerides in time of energy excess and breaks down triglycerides to release fatty acids and glycerol in times of fasting.

Insulin allows the entry of glucose into adipose tissue, where it helps mainly in the esterification of fatty acids into triglycerides and suppresses lipolysis. The release of fatty acids and glycerol by hydrolysis is stimulated by glucagon, growth hormone, ACTH, and the catecholamines, epinephrine, and norepinephrine. Cortisol, thyroxine, theophylline, caffeine, and autonomic innervation of the adipose tissue also contribute to the mobilization of fatty acid.

ASPECTS OF OBESITY

The very *definition of obesity* is in question. A simple statement, such as defining obesity as 20% overweight, would not take stature into account; comparing the percentile of height with the percentile of weight may lead to an error because of the wide variation of weight percentile at a given age compared to the percentile variation with height. A further improvement in the definition would use the easily available weight-for-height charts and conservatively state that obesity is a value over the 80th to 90th percentile. Formulas proposed to convert body weight to percentage of fat are generally suspect because they do not take into consideration the varying body types of children. The *weight-for-length index* (*WLI*) has been suggested as a valid formula in childhood. It a mathematically derived version of a weight-for-height chart and is calculated by the following:

$$WLI = A/B \text{ over } C/D \text{ times } 100.$$

A = child's weight
B = child's height
C = ideal 50th% weight for child's age
D = ideal 50th% height for child's age

A value of 90 to 109 is normal, a value of 110 to 119 is overweight, and a value over 120 is obese.

Triceps skin thickness measurement standards are available and objective, but most observers are unpracticed in the technique, many children complain about the pinching sensation, and a calipers is not always available in pediatric settings.

Indirect techniques, such as *underwater weighing*, will quantify body fat, but the apparatus is not readily available. The same problem occurs with the measurement of total body ^{40}K (present in nonadipose tissue), which requires a large gamma counter.

In fact, although the prejudices of the observer will come into play, it is usually obvious which child is subject to social pressure because of obesity after a casual glance and which child is only minimally chubby. Possibly, the more difficult step is to convince an oblivious (and often obese) parent that the child needs treatment for obesity or to dissuade an overcritical (and often thin) parent that the child is close enough to average to need no therapy.

Clinical Obesity

As a general rule, *organic obesity* combines short stature and obesity; *exogenous obesity* leads to advanced skeletal maturation and tall stature during childhood.

Organic Obesity and Short Stature

The much maligned *hypothyroidism* rarely causes extreme obesity in childhood. Most cases of hypothyroidism are chubby and have coarse features with short stature, delayed bone age, and high (immature) upper to lower segment ratios. A measure of protein binding of thyroid hormone must be obtained in addition to a measurement of serum thyroid hormone when evaluating a patient so that a child with thyroid binding protein deficiency will not be labeled falsely as hypothyroid.

Growth hormone deficient patients are described as cherubic due to their "rolly-polly" appearance of generalized increase in adipose tissue in the untreated state. They are, of course, short and grow poorly with an upper to lower segment ratio normal for bone age. They may experience hypoglycemia. The diagnosis is described in Chapter 1.

Patients with *pituitary-hypothalamic tumors* may combine growth hormone deficiency, thyroid deficiency, and gonadotropin deficiency, or any combination of these. The patients are often obese; and neurologic manifestations, including but not limited to headache and visual impairment, may be seen. Craniopharyngiomas or germinomas of the hypothalamus are the most common tumors in this age group, and the obesity may occur before or after diagnosis and surgical or radiation therapy. The archaic term Froehlich syndrome, or adiposo-genito-dystrophy, refers to a hypothalamic-pituitary tumor with obesity but was first applied to a patient with a tuberculous granuloma of the hypothalamic-pituitary area; the term is less than descriptive and no longer serves any function. There are a fascinating group of patients who grow well after craniopharyngioma removal, in spite of their growth hormone deficiency; they are obese.

The first manifestation of *Cushing syndrome* is cessation of growth, but weight gain is appreciated quickly and becomes profound. The pattern is truncal obesity with wasting thinness of the extremities. The "buffalo hump" at the back of the neck and stria may or may not appear; because they may be seen in exogenous obesity, stria do not strongly differentiate these children. The diagnosis is described in Chapter 4.

Pseudohypoparathyroidism and *pseudopseudohypoparathyroidism* present with a phenotype of a short stature, round face, short fourth and fifth metacarpals, and often mental developmental delay. The difference between the two is in the low serum calcium and high phosphorous concentrations, often with a history of seizures in pseudohypoparathyroidism and the normal values in pseudopseudo-hypoparathyroidism.

There are several syndromes of obesity and short stature that are diagnosed by the physical findings. The *Prader-Willi-Labhart syndrome* consists of short stature, obesity, insatiable hunger, infantile hypotonia, mental retardation, small hands and feet, and a characteristic face with almond-shaped eyes.   Behavior modification has been increasingly successful in such patients in controlling weight gain, and some residential facilities have had success as well. Growth hormone is said to have some beneficial effect on growth, but this treatment is presently experimental and only short-term data is available. Puberty often is delayed. We are aware of several cases in which the patients grew well in childhood (as would be expected in exogenous obesity, but due to advanced bone age had early epiphyseal fusion and achieved a short adult stature.) Some patients have abnormalities of chromosome 15, but the significance of this may be in question.

The *Laurence-Moon-Biedl syndrome* consists of short stature, obesity, retinitis pigmentosum and visual impairment, mental retardation, polydactyly in an autosomal recessive pattern. Puberty may be delayed.

The *Alstrom-Hallgren syndrome* includes retinal degeneration and nerve deafness and occasionally diabetes mellitus and acanthosis nigricans.

Organic Obesity and Tall Stature

Any of these syndromes which include hyperinsulinism as a feature will provide a tendency toward weight gain and increased statural growth unless the hypoglycemia is so severe as to interfere with nutrition. Thus, babies and children with the *Beckwith-Weideman syndrome* or *β-cell adenomas* will follow this pattern unless extirpation of the hypersecretory sections of pancreas is achieved.

Tumors or congenital anomalies of the *ventromedial hypothalamus* are rare but can impair the sense of satiety and lead to massive obesity. If control of hypothalamic factors and pituitary function is not effected, tall stature may occur; if growth hormone release is decreased, short stature will result. Uncontrolled rage attacks are reported in rare patients with hypothalamic disease in addition to massive obesity.

Exogenous Obesity

If the cause of obesity relates to diet or activity levels, we may consider it exogenous. There remains considerable controversy over the effects of *heredity* and *environment* in the development of obesity. Studies of twins and adoptive parents strongly suggest a genetic influence, but a genetic tendency toward obesity is fulfilled only by the dietary and exercise programs of the subject; no one is doomed to become obese even if a family tendency is present. Further, an already obese child does not necessarily become an obese adult; various workers have shown that only 14% of obese infants become obese adults (compared to 6% of normals), 41% of obese 7 year olds become obese adults, and about 70% of obese 10-13 year olds become obese adults. Thus the older the child, the more likely that the obesity will become a chronic problem. It is generally accepted that obese persons engage in less activity than thinner persons; this pattern does not stand up to analysis, and even when it is found to be true, it is not clear that lack of activity caused the obesity or if the obesity caused a decrease in activity. Obese children are always thought to eat more than thin children but analysis of diet does not always bear this out either; the same diet seems able to cause obesity in one child but not in another of the same age and height. Thus, because of differences between subjects, it may be said that an obese child eats too much and exercises too little to allow a normal weight to result; the descriptor "too" may not apply to another child. The method of treatment is obvious: decrease caloric intake and increase energy expenditure. The means to achieve this goal is certainly not so obvious.

Metabolic concomitants in childhood exogenous obesity include *insulin resistance* and some degree of *carbohydrate intolerance* (but rarely adult-type diabetes mellitus), suppression of *growth hormone secretion* in response to secretagoges, and *elevated plasma lipid concentrations* for age.

Physical changes associated with obesity include a tendency toward advanced skeletal development, tall stature with early onset of puberty so that there is no resulting increase in adult height, an increased incidence of slipped capital femoral epiphyses. In boys, gynecomastia may appear more severe at the time of puberty, and at all ages the fat pad over the mons pubis may hide the base of the penis and falsely suggest hypogonadism. Girls with obesity may have significant insulin resistance associated with acanthosis nigricans; virilization may occur with enlargement of the clitoris.

Social effects of obesity include a sense of isolation, poor self-image, and depression; these same factors may be said to predispose to obesity as well as to result from it.

As noted above, the *perception of obesity* will vary due to social class, educational level, and ethnic group. However, whatever the perception of the surrounding group, a person will be evaluated by the perceptions of the society as a whole, and society has been taught by books, magazines, movies, and the ever-present television that obese people are likely to be lazier, messier, and often less bright than thinner people and are the appropriate target of jokes: we are a weightist society. For example, obese girls were accepted at a far lower rate to a college than thin girls with the same grade point averages; the results of job recruitment often follow the same pattern.

The media not only shapes our view of obesity but may cause obesity. Television watching decreases time for vigorous activity, and there is a positive relationship between television viewing and weight gain in childhood. Further, a child watching television will see something in the order of 5 to 10 episodes of eating per hour with no demonstrable effect on the weight of the person eating; commercials during the shows most often watched by children and adolescents commonly feature candy bars and sugar-laced cold drinks alternating with stylish and often tight preteen and teenage clothing. Eating while watching television is a national sport.

Treatment of Obesity

The older child or teenager with obesity often will have a negative self-image derived from peers and parents. An obesity treatment program should not be so coercive that if the program fails the subjects will have intensified negative feelings. In a situation in which motivation of patient and parent is low, it is not appropriate to initiate a treatment program until at least the child is ready. Younger children are at the mercy of the diet given to them by caregivers and family, many of whom may not know how to set limits and may regularly reward the child with food. Older teenagers reaching the stage of increased independence can some-times achieve weight control even without the compliance of their family, although the course is much easier with cooperation of all involved.

It may be useful first to mention what is not useful in the treatment of obesity. Maintaining a strict diet, such as those found in hundreds of books, cannot help because the child is not taught how to deal with the cafeteria of food choices that will be encountered after the diet ends, as it must; binge eating may be triggered by and follow restrictive diets. Weight loss may be detrimental for a growing child, and rapid weight loss, such as is found in advertisements in newspapers and magazines for diets, is usually unobtainable and can be downright dangerous; maintaining a stable weight while the stature increases is preferable in all but the most massive obesity in childhood. Dietary substitutes and particularly powdered diet drinks are not proved safe for children and may lack nutrient balance, not to mention that, in some cases, they have been shown to be dangerous in adults. There is no present role for anorexigenic drug therapy or surgery (stapling, intestinal bypass, or liposuction) in the treatment of obesity in childhood or adolescence. Commercial weight loss programs may emphasize one aspect, such as dieting, without including an analysis of the family situation that reinforces abnormal eating patterns.

What is useful is a program that offers education about nutritive values of food, understands the psychology of childhood and adolescence, emphasizes the development of habits of movement and exercise that may be carried through life, gently invokes support of weight loss by individual counseling or group sessions, and modifies that behavior that stimulates non-necessary eating. Thus, there is a good chance that a pattern of living compatible with normal weight can be instilled by teaching the subject that french fries are highly caloric but carrot or celery sticks can be eaten with impunity; that habit, boredom, or depression drives the craving for candy or other foods outside of normal meals; and that moderate exercise with friends can be pleasurable rather than a chore. Parental involvement through parallel sessions or individual counseling has been shown to increase the success of a program. Such programs are noted in the reference list and may be available in university or clinical settings in various locations across the country; school-based programs of prevention that include exercise and nutrition information would be the ideal recourse, but they are rarely available due to personnel or funding limitations or lack of appreciation of the problem of childhood obesity.

Patients in dysfunctional families in which unresolved conflicts and unstated tension is the rule will benefit from family therapy, if it is accepted, before any concentration is made upon the obese child. Thus, a family assessment is mandatory before any weight control program is attempted. A patient who manifests severe depression is not usually appropriate for the customary group treatment programs; individual psychotherapy is indicated in such a situation.

Suggested Readings

Abraham S, Collin C, Nordsieck M: Relationship of child weight status to morbidity to adults. Public Health Rep 1970;86:273

Av-Ruskin TW, Pillai S, Kasi K, et al: Decreased prolactin secretion in childhood obesity. J Pediatr 1985;106:373

Berkowitz RI, Agras WS, Korner AF, et al: Physical activity and adiposity: A longitudinal study from birth to childhood. J Pediatr 1985;106:734

Charney M et al: Childhood antecedents of adult obesity. N Engl J Med 1976;295:6

Epstein LH, Wing RR, Valoski A: Childhood obesity. Pediatr Clin North Am 1985;32:363

Mellin L: Shapedown; Weight Management Program for Adolescents. San Francisco: Balboa Pub, 1983

Richards GE, Cavallo A, Meyer WJ, et al: Obesity, acanthosis nigricans, insulin resistance and hyperandrogenism: Pediatric perspective and natural history. J Pediatr 1985;107:893

Stark K, et al: Longitudinal study of obesity in the National Survey of Health and Development Br Med J 1981;283:12

Wexman M, Stunkard AJ: Caloric intake and expenditure of obese boys. J Pediatr 1980;96:187

Chapter 12

Endocrine Emergencies

HYPOGLYCEMIA

Hypoglycemia may be heralded by adrenergic symptoms and neurologic symptoms. Thus, sweatiness, shakiness, and tachycardia will occur due to norepinephrine and epinephrine, whereas decreased mentation and stupor and even coma will be mediated by neurologic mechanisms; seizures may occur if the drop in glucose is abrupt and great. The neonate may not be able to mount such responses, and decreased activity, poor feeding, and lethargy may be the sum of indications of hypoglycemia.

The treatment of hypoglycemia initially will be sugar administration. If the symptoms are mild, oral table sugar or sweet liquids may be offered. In cases where the patient is combative or uncooperative, it is possible to administer the sugar on the buccal mucosa in the form of jelly or honey (honey should only be given to children over one year of age due to the possibility of infant botulism) to avoid the possibility of aspiration. If no intravenous line is available, a dose of intramuscular glucagon (0.03mg/kg up to 1 mg) can be used to increase blood sugar concentrations quickly in patients expected to have adequate glycogen stores.

Intravenous glucose is the optimal treatment in other cases and especially in neonates. It is important to administer solutions close to isotonic concentrations. There is no excuse for the use of undiluted 50% dextrose in a child, and even 25% dextrose is too concentrated in most cases. Rather, 12.5% dextrose can be given in a bolus of 1 to 2 ml/kg body weight as an acute measure. In cases of hyperinsulinism, there may be a rebound hypoglycemic episode after a bolus so a gradual weaning regime is indicated when discontinuing

160

therapy, rather than an acute "cold turkey" termination of the infusion. If the diagnosis of hyperinsulinism is entertained, a chronic glucose infusion is the next step after acutely stabilizing the glucose concentration. D10%/w at 8 to 10 mg/kg/min is an appropriate initial infusion rate, with adjustments based upon the clinical response (thus, 0.1 ml/kg/min will equate to 10 mg/kg/min). Obviously, appropriate sodium chloride and potassium must be given if there is likelihood of a long-term infusion. Further, the chronic infusion of glucose will cause a decrease in serum inorganic phosphate which may impair the function of 2,3-Diphosphoglycerate; monitoring of serum PO_4 is advised. The symptoms of hypoglycemia usually are easily reversible unless postictal depression results from a seizure (see Chapter 10).

HYPERGLYCEMIA

Usually, elevated blood sugar will occur associated with diabetes mellitus, but medication (e.g., diazoxide) or metabolic diseases also can cause this. Treatment of the underlying disorder will be curative. Insulin is administered according to the plan in Chapter 9 in patients with diabetes (see Chapter 9).

HYPERCALCEMIA

Hypercalcemia is far less common in childhood than in adults, particularly since the humoral hypercalcemia of malignancy is very rare in children. The symptoms of hypercalcemia very much depend on the degree of hypercalcemia with most patients with levels below 11.5 to 12 mg/dl being asymptomatic. The symptoms are lethargy, weakness, inability to concentrate mentally, and depression. Many patients have nausea, vomiting, anorexia, constipation, and weight loss. The QT interval on the electrocardiogram (EKG) may shorten and serve as an early indication of hypercalcemia. Because a high extracellular calcium concentration impairs the capacity of the distal tubule to respond to antidiuretic hormone, hypercalcemic patients have polyuria and an inability to concentrate the urine. If serum calcium rises to more than 16 mg/dl, stupor and coma may develop.

Good hydration is an essential requirement in promoting calciuria and the infusion of sodium chloride (at one and one-half to two times maintenance) is helpful. The administration of furosemide (1 to 2 mg/kg) has been suggested to increase urinary calcium excretion, but it may be risky: it must be emphasized that the patient is already likely to be dehydrated due to polyuria, and the furosemide must be counteracted by increased saline infusion to avoid severe dehydration and shock. Thiazide diuretics may increase serum calcium and should not be used. Glucocorticoid in pharmacologic doses (prednisone at 1 to 2 mg/kg) can reduce intestinal calcium absorption, but the effect will not occur for several days. Oral phosphate preparations will bind calcium in the intestine, but since phosphate leads to diarrhea there may be increased complications of fluid balance; further, deposition of calcium phosphate may occur in the soft tissues. Calcitonin is rarely necessary in pediatric patients, but it will exert an effect within an hour if given at a dose of 10 units/kg intravenously. If the cause of the hypercalcemia is hyperparathyroidism, an emergency parathyroidectomy is indicated (see Chapter 7).

HYPOCALCEMIA

Hypocalcemia can cause symptoms at different serum calcium concentrations in circumstances that change the ionized calcium concentration; for instance, in alkalosis, symptoms occur at a relatively higher calcium concentration than in acidosis, and patients with low serum protein concentrations are likely to be less symptomatic than those with normal protein concentrations. Symptoms of hypocalcemia are due to neuromuscular irritability and include muscle cramps, paresthesias, weakness, lethargy, and tetany or convulsions. Chvostek's, Trousseau's and the peroneal signs may be noted. It is only the more severe neurologic symptoms and signs that require emergency treatment. Chronic therapy is described in Chapter 7.

Intravenous infusion of 10% calcium gluconate at a dose of 50 to 200 mg/kg under EKG monitoring is an appropriate treatment of acute symptomatic hypocalcemia. This should be given slowly over 1 to 2 hours to avoid bradycardia. Infiltration of this substance can cause skin sloughing and necrosis and calcification of the area. If the cause of the hypocalcemia is hypomagnesemia, the appropriate therapy is administration of magnesium; 0.2 ml/kg of 50% magnesium sulfate can be given intramuscularly every 8 to 12 hours (see Chapter 7).

HYPOADRENAL SHOCK

Hypoadrenocorticism should be suspected in a patient with known Addison disease or congenital adrenal hyperplasia, with hypoglycemic and/or hypotensive crisis, with ambiguous genitalia or a boy with undescended testes, or with a family history of unexplained death in young siblings. Suggestive laboratory findings will include low serum glucose, low sodium accompanied by a high potassium (do not be fooled by a fallacious elevation of potassium due to hemolysis); confirmatory samples for the analysis of cortisol and precursors, depending on the clinical appearance, should be obtained before therapy is offered. Electrocardiographic monitoring is important while waiting for the return of the serum potassium; cardiac arrest is possible with elevated serum potassium and a high, peaked T wave may provide evidence that emergency efforts are necessary (such as the use of kayexelate resin).

Glucose is a mainstay of therapy in any type of hypoadrenalism; D5%/w or D10%/w are usually sufficient to raise the blood sugar. The administration of glucocorticoid cannot hurt a patient with suspected hypoadrenalism and can be given intravenously as hydrocortisone sodium succinate at a dose of 10 to 25 mg for a neonate and 50 to 100 mg for older children. If there is suspicion or knowledge of salt loss, sodium chloride should be administered in normal saline combined with the dextrose. In the past, intramuscular preparation of desoxycorticosterone acetate (DOCA) was available to help in the therapy of a salt losing emergency, but at the time of this writing is not available (see Chapter 2 and 4).

PHEOCHROMOCYTOMA

The symptoms of pheochromocytoma include flushing, tachycardia and hypertension and the latter two may present a medical emergency. Alpha adrenergic block should be administered before beta adrenergic blockade. Phenoxybenzamine is given orally (5 to 10 mg every 12 hours with increasing dosage until high blood pressure is controlled) for chronic therapy; intravenous or intramuscular phentolamine (1 mg per dose) is used for hypertensive crises which may occur while phenoxybenzamine is establishing its block. Beta blockade by propranolol (5 to 10mg given three to four times per day orally) is added when the heart rate rises as the alpha adrenergic blockade is being established; propranolol may cause paradoxical hypertension if given before the alpha adrenergic block is established. If the therapy above is ineffective, alphamethyltyrosine (a tyrosine hydroxylase inhibitor) can be started at 5 to 10 mg/kg/day given four times per day. Surgical preparation also includes administration of salt to repair the plasma volume, which is invariably low. The chronic treatment and surgical preparation for pheochromocytomas are described in Chapter 4.

AMBIGUOUS GENITALIA

Although it is not an immediately life threatening emergency, the appearance of a neonate with ambiguous genitalia presents a true psychosocial emergency. The way the condition is explained to the parents may mean the difference between comfortable acceptance of the baby and long-term disturbances of parent-child relationships and, ultimately, maladjustment of the child. A full discussion is found in Chapter 2, but a few reminders are appropriate.

No child should have gender assigned until an appropriate diagnosis is made; thus, obstetrician, pediatrician, family practitioner, and nurse should not hazard a guess in an effort to calm the family unless the disorder is identified and the decision on sex of rearing is made. It is never appropriate to refer to a patient as half-boy and half-girl, although physicians have done so. Diagnostic methods are changing in this field, and many texts and handbooks may be out of date; in this condition, above all, the assistance of a physician experienced with discussing disorders of sexual differentiation with the family and, in fact, experienced with the complexities of the diagnostic method is invaluable (see Chapter 2).

THYROTOXICOSIS-THYROID STORM

Thyroid storm consists of acute onset of hyperthermia and tachycardia in a patient with underlying hyperthyroidism; it is far rarer in childhood than in the adult patient. Precipitating factors are surgery, infection, and diabetic ketoacidosis. Symptoms include high fever, sweating, tachycardia and reduced mental state ranging from confusion to coma. Immediate therapy is indicated for this severe condition.

Propranolol (5 to 10 mg every six hours as a starting dose) can control some symptoms of hyperthyroidism. Propranolol can be given intravenously at a dose of 0.1 mg/kg up to a total of 5 mg, but an intra-atrial pacing catheter is a necessary precaution. Dexamethasone in a doses of 1 to 2 mg every 6 hours can lower serum T_3. Intravenous NaI in a dose of 1 to 2 grams per day may decrease the release of thyroid hormone from the thyroid gland; Lugol's solution can be given orally if the patient is conscious. A cooling blanket can help control the hyperpyrexia. Propylthiouracil will not take effect for several days, but to plan for the possibly extended course of the disorder, 200 to 300 mg can be given every six hours by slurry, if necessary. Fluid management must be watched and, if tachycardia causes heart failure, digitalis may be necessary (see Chapter 6).

CONGENITAL HYPOTHYROIDISM

Treatment of congenital hypothyroidism should begin when the diagnosis is established; as mentioned above, confirmatory tests beyond the neonatal screening tests must be obtained. In those cases where the screening results show an extremely low T_4 and high TSH, treatment can be started before the confirmatory results are available, as it will be most unlikely that a mistake in diagnosis has occurred. Presently, recommended dosage of synthetic thyroxine is 10 μg/kg for the newborn (a dose of 25 μg is the usual daily dose in term newborns) and 2 to 5 μg/kg per day after one year of age with an eventual total dose of 100 to 150 μg at the maximum in a teenager. Thyroxine is most widely available in tablets and is crushed and administered in a small amount of formula or applesauce. Liquid thyroxine is available for parenteral use but is quite expensive; it has been used for patients who are unable to take medications orally (see Chapter 6).

Chapter 13

Dynamic Endocrine Tests and Laboratory Values

Dynamic tests of endocrine function are based on the physiologic control of the systems tested. The explanation of the physiology of the respective organs is explained at the beginning of the chapters dealing with those organs and, in many cases, the tests are discussed along with the physiology. This chapter is meant to be a summary of the various tests available, the "recipe" for their performance, and cautions about the pitfalls in the tests.

Usually, tests requiring several blood samples are performed with an indwelling catheter so that multiple samples can be obtained without multiple venopunctures. Quite often we have seen children tested by laboratories accustomed to dealing with adults; some children have had 10 to 15 venopunctures over a three hour period because the laboratory was not prepared to start an intravenous infusion. The intravenous fluid must be normal or one-half normal saline without dextrose so that there will be no tendency to clot the needle or catheter. Tests are best performed in the morning after an overnight fast except for water. It has been shown that a combination of tests can be performed at once (e.g., thyrotropin releasing factor (TRF), gonadotropin releasing hormone (GnRH), clonidine or L-dopa), but in a small child this may lead to the acute loss of too much blood, and the combined side effects of TRF and L-dopa or clonidine may lead to excessive nausea.

The tests are only as good as the laboratories where the samples are sent. Some laboratories geared toward adult samples will request very large samples that are not advisable on multiple sampling in a child. They may have standards only for adult values so that the numbers reported for children are inaccurate for the pediatric range; this is most common in sex steroid values.

Many tests of endocrine function can be interpreted only in comparison with another measurement. For instance, insulin must be matched to glucose, parathyroid hormone to calcium, and vasopressin to osmolality. The measurement of an isolated endocrine value without its associated factor may not be informative, and on occasion may be misleading.

GROWTH HORMONE TESTING

A single growth hormone determination is of no use except in the rare case of pituitary gigantism or Laron dwarfism! This is probably the most misunderstood point in the diagnosis of growth hormone deficiency. Further, because of variation in response in any dynamic test, it is important to "bracket" the time at which you expect the peak to occur with samples taken at 15 to 30 minute intervals. Lastly, it should be appreciated that, because of individual variations in response, more than one pharmacologic test of growth hormone secretion is necessary to prove classic growth hormone deficiency; a normal response of growth hormone greater than 10ng/ml in any test is considered normal in most laboratories and eliminates the diagnosis of classic growth hormone deficiency. It must be recalled that there are children who require growth hormone for improved growth but who will respond to the tests with perfectly normal results.

Ten minutes after 10 minutes of vigorous *exercise* (almost to the point of exhaustion) 80% of normal children will raise their growth hormone concentrations.

Sequential samples at night may be taken in the hope that the peak that customarily occurs 90 minutes after the onset of sleep is captured, but this method is inconvenient in most hospitals.

Sampling for growth hormone levels every 10 to 15 minutes for 24 or 12 hours has been suggested as a way to determine if a normal *circadian rhythm* of growth hormone secretion is present; however, few hospitals are able to perform such a test, and the personnel to perform this are generally unavailable except in a research setting. The benefit of such testing over conventional secretogogue testing is unproven.

Secretogogues invoked in the testing for growth hormone deficiency are given the first thing in the morning after an over-night fast. The child may drink water, but any sugar or fat may decrease the response to growth hormone testing. Obesity will dull the response to growth hormone testing and tests in obese patients may be difficult to interpret. Two tests usually are performed because in many cases a normal child can fail to raise growth hormone concentration after one test.

L-Dopa in doses of 125 mg for body weight up to 15 kg, 250 mg for weight up to 35 kg, and 500 mg for body weight over 35 kg is given and samples taken at 0, 30, 60, and 90 minutes; nausea and vomiting are possible side effects which may occur for a few hours after administration.

Clonidine in a dose of 0.1 to 0.15 mg/m^2 can be given at the same time samples as noted for L-dopa; side effects may be a degree of hypotension and lethargy lasting for several hours.

Arginine intravenous infusion of 0.5gm/kg body weight up to 20 g over 20 minutes can be given to test for growth hormone secretion with samples taken at the same times as above; no side effects are likely.

Insulin-induced hypoglycemia (after 0.075 to 0.1 units/kg body weight of intravenous insulin) is an effective but potentially dangerous test; the patient must be shown to have a normal fasting blood sugar (>70 mg/dl) just before the test, must not have a known tendency towards hypoglycemia or seizures, a patent intravenous line must be available to infuse dextrose should a hypoglycemic seizure occur, and the patient must be watched carefully by a physician during the test. If severe hypoglycemia occurs, dextrose must be administered, but no more than 25% dextrose at 1 ml/kg should be infused so that a rise in blood sugar will occur but no severe change in serum osmolality results. Glucose and growth hormone should be measured at 0, 15, 20, 30, 60, 90 minutes and cortisol at 60 and 90 minutes if this test is performed for evaluation of ACTH reserve as well as GH reserve.

GHRH is available for clinical research projects but is not yet in general use. A dose of 5 to 10 µg/kg is administered by an intravenous bolus and blood samples obtained for GH analysis over the following hour. Those patients with abnormal responses may demonstrate no rise in GH during the test or an impaired rise in GH after GHRH; it is not yet clear what causes the differing responses between subjects. The GHRH test has helped the elucidation of many aspects of growth hormone physiology but does not yet appear to offer a major improvement over conventional testing plans.

Previously, children often were primed with *propranolol* or, if prepubertal, with *testosterone* or *estrogen* for boys and girls, respectively, to increase the likelihood of a normal response to secretogogue testing. Because of increased availability of growth hormone and doubts as to what the true cutoff of normal growth hormone response is in an individual, most pediatric endocrinologists no longer prime the subjects and accept the unprimed test results in the decision of whether to treat with growth hormone or not (see Chapter 1).

THYROTROPIN RELEASING HORMONE TESTING

A dose of 200μg of TRF is given intravenously and thyroid-stimulating hormone (TSH) measured at 0, 10, 15, 30, 60, 90, 120, 180 minutes. A normal response is a rise in TSH of 10 to 40 mIU/ml after about 15 minutes, whereas in secondary hypothyroidism there will be no rise in TSH; in tertiary hypothyroidism the rise will be delayed until 60 to 120 minutes and the TSH may continue to rise during the 180 minute period. There will be no rise in TSH after TRF with the autonomous thyroxine secretion characteristic of Graves' disease (see Chapter 6).

CALCITONIN TESTING

There are several provocative tests for calcitonin secretion in diagnosing the presence of a medullary carcinoma of the thyroid; some patients will respond to one or the other of the calcium or pentagastrin tests so that the combined test is preferable and has been determined to have fewer false negatives. To perform these tests: calcium gluconate in a dose of 15 mg of elemental calcium per kg of body weight can be infused over four hours and calcitonin determined at baseline, three and four hours; pentagastrin at a dose of 0.5 μg/kg can be infused as an intravenous bolus over 5 to 10 seconds and calcitonin measured at 0, 2, and 3 minutes; a combined calcium/ pentagastrin test requires the intravenous administration of 2mg/kg of elemental calcium over 50-60 seconds followed by the dose of pentagastrin noted above. Some laboratories report that the presence of medullary carcinoma of the thyroid requires (1) a basal concentration of calcitonin below 200 pg/ml, which increases to greater than 300 pg/ml after a combined calcium/pentagastrin test or (2) if the basal level of calcitonin is greater than 300 pg/ml(and less than 600), the calcium/pentagastrin test should cause a fivefold rise in calcitonin. *Note that different laboratories have different standards for this test; the laboratory must be consulted before interpreting the results (see Chapter 6).*

GONADOTROPIN RELEASING FACTOR TESTING

A 100 μg bolus of GnRH is administered intravenously and serum samples are taken at 0, 10, 15, 30, 60, 90, 120 minutes to be analyzed for LH and FSH. A rise of LH greater than 16 mIU/ml occurs in pubertal or adult subjects, whereas a far smaller rise is found in prepubertal subjects; thus, the rise in LH after GnRH is a useful reflection of pubertal status. There is some variation in response, so that a pubertal response is not a guarantee that a patient will progress through puberty or that a girl will have regular menstrual periods. Girls of all ages release more FSH than boys so that the FSH response to GnRH is not an adequate reflection of pubertal state (see Chapter 3).

TESTICULAR TESTING

If a patient has cryptorchism or if it is desired to determine the ability of the testes to produce adequate testosterone, testicular stimulation is appropriate. The administration of human chorionic gonadotropin (hCG), 3000 units/m^2 intramuscularly, should induce a rise in testosterone over 100 ng/dl within 72 hours in a cryptorchid patient; if the patient is in midchildhood or older, one injection of hCG may not be adequate to stimulate the quiescent Leydig cells. If hCG is given three times per week for two weeks, the testes may descend into the scrotum if the inguinal ring is not definitively too small; it is useful to measure serum testosterone 24 hours after the last injection of hCG to see if testosterone secretion can be induced over a longer period of time (see Chapters 2 and 3).

ADRENOCORTICAL-ADRENAL TESTING

The *low-dose dexamethasone suppression* test utilizes 1.25 mg/m^2 of dexamethasone divided into four doses per day for two days; if the urinary 17-OHCs on the second day of the test fall 50% from the two baseline collections (or if the 17-OHCS is less than 1mg/m^2 and the urine free cortisol less than 25 μg/m^2), the patient is likely to have exogenous obesity. We find it useful to collect serum adrenocorticotropic hormone (ACTH) and cortisol concentrations during the baseline and dexamethasone suppression phases of the test to see if serum values are also affected (e.g., if the cortisol is less than 5 μg/dl or the serum ACTH is less than 25 pg/ml).

In the *high-dose dexamethasone suppression test*, 3.75mg/m^2 of dexamethasone is divided into four doses per day, given for two days and urinary 17-OHCs on the second day is compared to the two baseline collections; in Cushing disease there will be complete suppression of urinary 17-OHCs, whereas in the ectopic ACTH syndrome or with autonomous cortisol secretion, there will be no suppression over baseline levels.

To test for ACTH reserve, *insulin-induced hypoglycemia* may be used if the cautions noted under growth hormone testing with insulin are heeded.

Another useful test of the ACTH-adrenal axis is the *ACTH stimulation test*. In the morning between 8:00 to 9:00 AM, after a fast except for water, a blood sample is drawn for cortisol (and ACTH if it has not been determined earlier in the workup), a bolus of 250 μg synthetic ACTH (usually 1-24 Cortrosyn but never intact natural ACTH) is given and after one hour, a blood sample is drawn for cortisol (or, if the test is performed for the diagnosis of a congenital adrenal hyperplasia, 17OHP, DHA, progesterone or other appropriate metabolites). In primary adrenal failure, the baseline cortisol will be low and will not rise after ACTH; in ACTH or CRF deficiency, the cortisol will rise 10 to 20 μg/dl; in the normal subject cortisol will rise to over 25 μg/dl. In disorders of the 21 hydroxylase enzyme, a normal person will have a rise in 17 OHP to 100 to 300 ng/dl; a patient with classical 21 OH deficiency will have a rise to over 10,000 ng/dl; a patient with late onset or cryptic 21 OH deficiency will have a rise to 2000 to 10,000 ng/dl and heterozygotes for any form of the 21 OH deficiencies will have a rise falling between normals and classic 21 OH deficiency, between 200 to 2000 ng/dl.

A *metyrapone test* will reveal ACTH reserve by blocking negative feedback inhibition of cortisol upon ACTH secretion and thereby increase ACTH; the rise in ACTH is indicated by an increase in compound S, the substrate of the 11-hydroxylase enzyme that is temporarily blocked by metyrapone. A 30 mg/kg dose of metyrapone up to a maximum of 3 g is administered at midnight, and a blood sample is taken for Cortisol and 11-deoxycortisol (compound S) at 6:00 to 8:00 AM. In a valid test, a normal person will have a cortisol less than 5 μg/dl (proving that a block was established) and a compound S of more than 10 μg/dl. A patient with ACTH deficiency will have low cortisol and compound S (see Chapter 4).

ADRENAL MEDULLARY TESTING

Testing for pheochromocytoma is now carried out on urinary collections without stimulation, as the pharmacologic tests previously used (such as phentolamine, tyrosine, and histamine tests) have been shown to be dangerous and somewhat variable in their results (see Chapter 4).

PROLACTIN TESTING

The TRF test is performed as noted under thyroid testing, and a sample is obtained for prolactin at the same times as for TSH. A normal person will have a peak of prolactin of 10 to 50 ng/ml within 60 minutes; a person with hypothalamic dysfunction may have a far higher response, and those with severe pituitary deficiency will have no rise (see Chapter 3).

VASOPRESSIN TESTING

The cautions noted in Chapter 5 must be considered before a water deprivation test is performed. The child should have a normal dinner, and the usual nighttime routine should continue. The next morning the first voided urine should be analyzed for osmolality to determine whether the child even needs a test; if the urine osmolality is elevated, the child apparently is able to concentrate the urine appropriately. If the test is indicated, body weight and blood pressure should be determined, and a serum sodium and a hematocrit should be obtained. At that time a normal breakfast can be given with normal fluid and then all oral intake should cease. Weight and blood pressure should be taken hourly, serum osmolality as well as hematocrit every two hours, and all urine volume monitored and osmolality measured every void. The test should cease if the weight drops 5%, the blood pressure falls, or the osmolality rises above 300 mosm/liter. Otherwise, at the end of eight hours the serum and urine osmolality should be compared and a serum vasopressin obtained to match with the osmolalities (the vasopressin value will not return for weeks from the laboratory but may prove useful if the diagnosis is still in doubt). A patient with diabetes insipidus cannot concentrate the urine to more than 1.5 times the serum osmolality so that if the serum osmolality rises to 300 mosm/liter or higher the urine should be more than 450 mosm/liter.

In an intermediate situation where a trend toward dehydration is developing, a continuation of the thirst may be necessary. Further, in partial diabetes insipidus a patient may pass one test with adequate urinary concentration; however, if the test is repeated the next day, the patient may be totally unable to concentrate the urine because of the exhaustion of the patient's meager supply of vasopressin. If the serum osmolality has risen without an increase of urine osmolality, a dose of aqueous vasopressin is administered at 0.3 ml/m^2 of 20 units/ml aqueous vasopressin subcutaneously or 0.05 to 0.15 ml of DDAVP in a nostril. In the next 30 to 60 minutes the volume of urine and the concentration is compared to the values before the exogenous vasopressin or DDAVP. In central diabetes insipidus, at the end of the thirst, maximal but inadequate endogenous vasopressin already has been released so that the exogenous vasopressin will further concentrate the urine. If the patient has psychogenic polydipsia, because of the excess water load the patient has taken in prior to the onset of the test, the serum osmolality will not rise above normal during the thirst; if the patient has maintained an adequate medullary interstitial gradient in spite of high urine flow, the exogenous vasopressin will cause further concentration of the urine. A patient with nephrogenic diabetes insipidus will not be able to concentrate urine in spite of rising serum osmolality and with the addition of exogenous vasopressin will not further raise urine osmolality or reduce urine volume (see Chapter 5).

GLYCEMIC TESTING

There is little reason for a glucose tolerance test in the diagnosis of diabetes mellitus or hypoglycemia, as random samples for blood sugar that are over 200 mg/dl are diagnostic in the presence of symptoms. On occasion, however, this test may be useful, for instance in the differential diagnosis of type I vs type II diabetes mellitus (DM) or in the investigation of a potential hyperinsulinemic state. The test must be performed after three days on a high carbohydrate diet (50% of calories as carbohydrates with a large diet for weight); the test should not be performed within weeks of an illness. After an overnight fast, an intravenous infusion is started, and oral glucose in a dose of 1.75 gm/kg up to a maximum of 75 g is given in a no more than 25% solution. Blood samples are obtained for glucose (use fluoride-containing tubes or ensure that the analyses will be performed quickly after the blood is drawn) and insulin at 0, 30, 60, 90, 120, 180, 240, and 300 minutes. Urine is collected along with the blood samples as possible and analyzed for sugar.

Elevated blood sugar concentrations of greater than 120 mg/dl (or plasma sugar >140mg/dl) while fasting or 120 mg/dl of blood sugar (or >140mg/dl of plasma sugar) at two hours is considered an impaired response suggestive of diabetes mellitus in the presence of customary symptoms. The absence of appropriate insulin secretion in the presence of glucose intolerance demonstrates type I DM while an insulin response would suggest insulin resistance characteristic of type II DM (see Chapters 9 and 10).

A COMPENDIUM OF LABORATORY VALUES
USEFUL IN PEDIATRIC ENDOCRINOLOGY

Laboratory values may vary with the laboratory performing the test, in spite of standardization procedures. This list is meant only as a guide. The laboratory performing the test should be consulted for exact standards. Also, remember the cautionary note above, that only laboratories experienced in pediatric procedures should be used. A pediatric laboratory is more likely to use less blood, a consideration of great importance in a complex young patient. Also, a pediatric laboratory is more likely to give accurate values than a laboratory mainly interested in adult diseases when measuring hormones that rise with development, such as the sex steroids; the difference between a testosterone value of 10 and 40 ng/dl may be of great importance in a boy undergoing evaluation for delayed puberty but may be of no importance in an adult evaluated for impotence. An adult laboratory may report a value as 60 ng/dl when they actually can measure only to less than 60 ng/dl. This distinction is of great value in a developing adolescent patient who has a true testosterone concentration of 20 ng/dl but who has a reported value of 60 ng/dl because of the reasons noted. Many values are given in relation to the stage of development or age range in which the values are found.

Note that many hormone values cannot be interpreted unless linked to their regulatory factor: insulin and glucose, parathyroid hormone and calcium, ACTH and cortisol, and vasopressin and osmolality are only a few examples.

All values are given for fasting serum unless otherwise noted. All 24-hour values must be measured on full 24-hour urine specimens or the test may be meaningless; e.g., if a morning six-hour collection for cortisol is sent as a representative sample and multiplied by four for the whole 24 hours, the results will be fallaciously high; if a nighttime sample is sent, the results may be fallaciously low!

The values that follow are taken from laboratory standards at University of California Davis Medical Center, Nichols Institute (with permission), references noted at the end of the preceding chapters as well as the texts noted at the end of this chapter. Values will vary according to laboratory and with improved techniques: *check the normal values in use at the time of the test for the laboratory which performs the tests.*

ADRENAL FUNCTION

Cortisol
  AM Cortisol   10-20 μg/dl
  PM Cortisol   5-12 μg/dl

24-hour urinary 17 OHCS   <4.5 mg/m^2

24-hour urinary 17 KS   infant over 1 week <3
                                     pubertal boy 5-15 mg
                                     pubertal girl 5-13 mg

24-hour urine free cortisol   <60 μg/m^2

ACTH
  AM ACTH   50-130 pg/ml
  PM ACTH   20-50 pg/ml

11-deoxycortisol (compound S)

                                 <1 μg/dl

17-hydroxyprogesterone   cord blood 1000-4000 ng/dl
                                     older age <150 ng/dl

Dehydroepiandrosterone-
sulfate   cord blood 50-250 μg/dl
                                     older age <60 μg/dl
                                     pubertal 60-500 μg/dl

Deoxycorticosterone   2-15 ng/ml

Corticosterone   70-800 ng/dl

Aldosterone   under 1 year 5-130 ng/dl
                                     1-4 years 5-60 ng/dl
                                     4-8 years 4-76 ng/dl
                                     8-12 years 3-28 ng/dl
                                     12-16 years 1-18 ng/dl
                                     all values for normal sodium diet
                                     and supine position

Plasma renin activity   3 months-1 year <15 ng/ml/hr
                                     1-4 years <10 ng/ml/hr
                                     4-15 years <6 ng/ml/hr
                                     supine adult .2-3 ng/ml/hr

Urinary norepinephrine   <1 year 10-70 μg/m^2
                                   >1 year 10-45 μg/m^2

Urinary epinephrine $1\text{-}10 \; \mu g/m^2$

Urinary VMA $1\text{-}3 \; mg/m^2$

Urinary HVA   1-2 years 3-25 μg/mg creat.
                              2-5 years 1-14 μg/mg creat.
                              5-18 years 1-10 μg/mg creat.
                              >18 years .2-3 μg/mg creat.

GROWTH HORMONE FUNCTION

Basal growth hormone   <2 ng/ml
(useless except for pituitary
gigantism or Laron's dwarfism)

Stimulated growth hormone   7-12 ng/ml

Somatomedin C or IGF-1   1-10 years .15-1/ U/ml
                              puberty 1-3 U/ml

GLYCEMIC FUNCTION

Glucose   55-120 mg/dl

Hemoglobin A1C   3.4-6.7 %

Glycosylated hemoglobin   3-6 %

Urinary glucose   negative

Insulin   <20 μU/ml (depending upon glucose)
                              nondetectable if hypoglycemic

C peptide   1-4 ng/ml

Insulin/glucose ratio   <0.5

ß hydroxybutyrate   1-5 mM

Acetoacetate   <1 mg/dl

Acetone   <1 mg/dl

Urine ketone bodies   negative

Pyruvate   .5-2 mg/ml

Lactate   5-20 mg/ml

GONADOTROPIN FUNCTION

Basal LH   prepubertal <4 mIU/ml
                                      pubertal 4-12 mIU/ml

GnRH stimulated LH   >15.6 mIU/ml

Basal FSH   prepubertal <4 mIU/ml
                                      pubertal 4-12 mIU/ml

hCG   <10 mIU/ml

OVARIAN FUNCTION

(total estrogens have no clear use in pediatric endocrinology and should not be ordered)

Estradiol

  in females   < 6 months <60 pg/ml
                                     older age <15 pg/ml
                                     pubertal 20-250 pg/ml
                                     (midcyle may reach 750 pg/ml)

  in males   prepubertal <15 pg/ml
                                     older ages < 15 pg/ml

Progesterone   prepubertal <2 ng/ml
                                     post-ovulatory >5 ng/ml

PARATHYROID FUNCTION

Total calcium   8.8-10.5 mg/dl

Ionized calcium   4.6-5.4 mg/dl

Parathyroid hormone

  N terminal   8-24 pg/ml

C terminal	50-330 pg/ml
25 OH vitamin D	10-40 ng/ml Southern California 15-55 ng/ml
1,25 OH vitamin D	20-60 pg/ml
Magnesium	1.6-2.6 mg/dl

PROLACTIN FUNCTION

Basal prolactin

prepubertal boys 3-12 ng/ml
pubertal boys 3-18 ng/ml
prepubertal girls 3-12 ng/ml
pubertal girls 3-25 ng/ml

TESTICULAR FUNCTION

Testosterone (T)

in boys

< 6 months < 100 ng/dl
older age < 15 ng/dl
pubertal 40-1000 ng/dl

in girls

prepubertal < 10 ng/dl
late pubertal < 30 ng/dl
adult < 70 ng/dl

Dihydrotestosterone(DHT)

in boys

cord blood < 50 ng/ml
prepubertal < 1 ng/dl
pubertal males 5-210 ng/dl

in girls

cord blood < 22 ng/ml
prepubertal < 1 ng/ml
adult 1-8.5 ng/ml

Androstenedione

prepubertal 10-50 ng/dl
pubertal males 50-240 ng/dl

Sex hormone binding globulin

in adult males

.2-1.4 ug DHT bound/dl

in adult non-pregnant females

.6-3.6 ug DHT bound/dl

THYROID FUNCTION

Thyroxine by RIA	cord blood 7-13 μg/dl 1-3 days of age 12-23 μg/dl older age 5.5-12 μg/ml
Triiodothyronine by RIA	cord blood 15-75 ng/dl 1-3 days 100-740 ng/dl older age 80-240 ng/dl
Resin T_3 uptake	0.85-1.15
Free thyroxine index (T_7)	older age 5-12
Free thyroxine	older age 1.5-4 ng/dl
Free T_3	older age 240-580 pg/dl
Thyroid binding globulin (TBG)	<1 year 1.5-5.4 mg/dl >1 year 1.2-3 mg/dl
Thyroid stimulating hormone (TSH)	<5 μU/ml
Ultrasensative TSH	0.7-5 μU/ml
Thyroid stimulating immunoglobulin	negative
Anti-microsomal antibodies	negative (<1:400)
Anti-thyroglobulin antibodies	negative (<1:100)
Calcitonin in males	basal <30 pg/ml after pentagastrin <110 pg/ml after Ca/pentagastrin <350 pg/ml
in females	basal <17 pg/ml after pentagastrin <30 pg/ml after Ca/pentagastrin <100 pg/ml

Thyroglobulin   childhood 20-50 ng/ml
                                 13-18 years 9-27 ng/ml

VASOPRESSIN FUNCTION

Arginine vasopressin   1-14 pg/ml

Serum osmolality   270-300 mosm/kg

Urine osmolality   50-1200 mosm/kg

Urine specific gravity   1.001-1.030

Suggested Readings

Greenspan FS, Forsham PH: Basic and Clinical Endocrinology. San Mateo, CA: Medical Publications, 1986

Kaplan SA: Clinical Pediatric and Adolescent Endocrinology. Philadelphia: WB Saunders, 1982

Nichols Institute: Pediatric Catalog. San Juan Capistrano, CA: Nichols Institute, 1986

Rudolph AM (editor): Pediatrics. Norwalk, CT: Appleton-Centrury-Crofts, 1982

Wilson JD, Foster DW (editors): Williams Textbook of Endocrinology 7th ed. Philadelphia: WB Saunders, 1985

Index